H O P E

Through Compassion and Despair

A SUPPORTER'S GUIDE TO ASSISTING
PERSONS WITH MENTAL ILLNESS

RENEE POLEY and BRENT POLEY

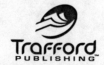

Trafford
PUBLISHING™

Hope, like the gleaming taper's light,
Adorns and cheers our way.
And still, as darker grows the night,
Emits a brighter ray.

OLIVER GOLDSMITH

Order this book online at www.trafford.com/07-0160
or email orders@trafford.com

Most Trafford titles are also available at major online book retailers.

Note for Librarians: A cataloguing record for this book is available from Library
and Archives Canada at www.collectionscanada.ca/amicus/index-e.html

Printed in Victoria, BC, Canada.

ISBN: 978-1-4251-1697-2

*We at Trafford believe that it is the responsibility of us all, as both individuals
and corporations, to make choices that are environmentally and socially sound.
You, in turn, are supporting this responsible conduct each time you purchase a
Trafford book, or make use of our publishing services. To find out how you are
helping, please visit www.trafford.com/responsiblepublishing.html*

*Our mission is to efficiently provide the world's finest, most comprehensive
book publishing service, enabling every author to experience success.
To find out how to publish your book, your way, and have it available
worldwide, visit us online at www.trafford.com/10510*

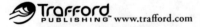 www.trafford.com

North America & international
toll-free: 1 888 232 4444 (USA & Canada)
phone: 250 383 6864 ♦ fax: 250 383 6804 ♦ email: info@trafford.com

The United Kingdom & Europe
phone: +44 (0)1865 722 113 ♦ local rate: 0845 230 9601
facsimile: +44 (0)1865 722 868 ♦ email: info.uk@trafford.com

10 9 8 7

CONTENTS

This book is dedicated to Brent whose struggle with Mental Illness and courage to face it touches my soul

FOREWORD

Over the years many people have approached me and shown great empathy and concern for my emotional health and well being. They have seen me go through numerous crises with Brent and his Mental Illness, and wondered how I could cope with it all. As difficult as it has been I have always held the philosophy of "there but for the grace of God go I", and never believed that any of my anguish could ever be compared to that of Brent's suffering.

This book is intended for those who show support to those loved ones in their lives who struggle with Mental Illness. As Supporters, whether we are family, friends, and/or community advocates, we can learn to take care of ourselves while we take care of others. Our unconditional love and support, as well as a practical approach to accessing and lobbying for required services, serve as the foundation for building community awareness and compassion for persons with disabilities.

—*Renee Poley*

READERS' COMMENTS

"As a caregiver, I found Chapter 2, One Cannot Turn Back the Hands of Time and Chapter 7, Letting Go, extremely helpful. I now live each day knowing I cannot change the things I have no control over, and that there is no magic formula to cure my daughter's Mental Illness. Unconditional love gives me the courage and strength to cope from day to day. Hope is always there!"

Donna, supporter of daughter
with bipolar condition

"Renee has captured, through the eyes of her remarkably brave son, Brent, many of the painful episodes of manic depression that he has experienced over the years. She has accomplished this primarily through her remarkable compassionate nature, while assisting him and others through their struggle with mental illness. I read this concise and very "reader-friendly" book, after being diagnoses as bipolar twenty-five years ago. Today, at sixty-seven years of age, while reading this book, I was able to recall some of my experiences as being similar to Brent's, for example, going without food and sleep, for days, yet continuing academic studies, on a post-graduate level.

Mental Illness is a chemical imbalance in the brain, causing us to experience "mood swings", and thus, the name, since the '60's, of "bipolar disorder". One day I can be "manic", the next "severely depressed" or vice versa. This can even occur within the same day, as I am a "rapid cycler" (a medical term). Bipolar disorder is said to be inherited through a gene that scientists have yet to pinpoint. Some Psychiatrists would also claim that there is an "environmental factor", which comes into play. This, certainly, was the case in my life. I wholeheartedly suggest you read this book written with clarity, humour and awareness of this very difficult human condition."

Rosemary Trainor,
person with bipolar condition

"Renee's writings of the different types of resources available in our community are the first I have seen; her writing of the role of support person and the methods of dealing with health professionals is detailed and extremely beneficial, and her writing of the Supporter as advocate, the Six Steps to Support, are very good too. Overall, her book was very touching to me and I thank her for writing it and letting me read it".

Laurie Atkinson,
person with bipolar condition.

"Renee Poley, along with her son, Brent, invites the reader to accompany them on a daring venture. They shine their bright light into the darkness and upon the heretofore masked and often frightening face of mental illness.

Throughout Poley's autobiographical account, we follow

Brent and his amazingly supportive family from his early years to manhood. We learn something of what it must be like to never be free from the specter that is bipolar illness: for it patiently sits in wait -intent upon stealing this bright mind and gentle soul away from those who love him. And though the disease we call 'bipolar' and/or 'manic-depression' is both elusive and cruel in the extreme, nevertheless, the Poleys' face their life-long challenge with determination, steadfastness, and yes, 'Hope'.

'Hope' is an apt title for Poley's work. Those who have a loved one suffering from Mental Illness will find in this book, a wealth of that commodity. One will also discover practical, straightforward directions through the baffling maze encountered on the path toward diagnosis, treatment, educational and employment options and social services.

I am pleased to note that 'compassion' is included in the title: compassion for the family member who is ill and compassion for those assuming the 'supporter' role. For, as illustrated throughout the book, those who are in the unenviable position of Supporter to a person experiencing Mental Illness need and deserve an intact support system to surround and uphold them.

Words like 'dignity', 'respect', 'compassion', and 'hope', outweigh, in my mind, the language of 'despair', and 'depression' in Poley's account. When that happens, the future for Persons with Mental Illness seems a little brighter.

Renee and Brent Poley triumph in their book, "Hope..." as they shine their light into the darkness and lead the way for others to follow.

I began to read "Hope..." one morning and found I

could not put it down. In the wee hours of the next day,
finally, I finished reading the book. I know it is one I will
on my bookshelf, to return to and reference, for many years
to come.

Eleanor Ryan, author,
Langley, B.C.

My Letter to God

Dear God, I write this letter
to tell you about our son;
please reach out and touch him,
and end his suffering.

He wanders down a distant road,
driven by racing thoughts;
Feeling the intensity of his high,
he reaches out to his brilliant sky.

He suffers from Mental Illness,
a curse he felt as a child;
the mania lurking within him,
makes his thoughts go wild.

He wants to work in society,
and earn his way through life;
please reach out and touch him,
and end his suffering.

Once he turned to street drugs,
and gambled what little he had;
shame and guilt they followed,
and made him feel so bad.

He suffers from Mental Illness,
Depression causes him deep pain;
when the angry shadow of darkness,
surrounds his soul again.

But he is strong, and he is kind,
and loyal to his friends;
please reach out and touch him,
and end his suffering.

Dear God, he keeps on trying,
to end his painful strife;
by efforts to manage his mood swings,
and improve the quality of his life.

He suffers from Mental Illness,
for that he's not blame,
please reach out and touch him,
and end his suffering.

Renee Poley

1

THE DAY IT ALL BEGAN

On February 7, 1968, an unusually warm and balmy day in Edmonton, my first child was born. My labor started late in the evening on February 6 while I was sitting in front of a typewriter, rushing to complete an English essay at the University of Alberta. I spoke to my unborn child, not knowing the sex at the time, and asked my baby to hang on until my essay was finished. I did nott know much about the process of giving birth as few books were available then on pregnancy and birthing, but I sensed that this was my time.

Brent came in to this world close to noon after a relatively short period of labor, although at the time, I felt it was the longest day of my life. When the Nurse handed him to me I was stunned by his huge, brown eyes as he stared right at me. There was one comment I overheard one Nurse making to another Nurse that left me feeling rather "unsettled", and stayed in the back of my mind for many years before I realized the significance of such a comment. As I held Brent close to me in the Hospital bed, I overheard "how unusual for his eyes to be wide open when he came out, and they are still that way". The word "unusual" frightened me but at the age of 20 years, and rather passive at the time towards the medical profession, I didn't have the courage to ask the Nurse what she meant by that comment. In fact, I felt rather annoyed; to me, Brent's big, brown eyes were breathtaking. He seemed so connected to me and as we looked at one another the rest of the world became a blur.

The Hospital stay lasted four days where I was allowed to rest and feed my baby every four hours until the Physician decided we could go home and begin our lives together. Standard procedure at that time was to keep a mother and her baby in the Hospital for several days which allowed me to rest and ask questions on how to care for my baby. The Nurses showed me how to feed, bath, change, and hold him during that time, as well as allow my body time to readjust and heal from the trauma of birthing.

During the first two days the Nurses expressed concern to me that my baby wasn't sleeping, and each time they brought him to me, he stared at me with those big, brown eyes. I couldn't understand why they were concerned as he seemed content and took to his bottle eagerly. Finally, one Nurse explained to me that they may have to give him sleeping medication as he needed to sleep. Shortly after her comment my baby had developed a normal sleeping pattern by the time we were discharged. To this day, I am unsure as to whether or not they gave him medication to help him sleep.

As a new mother, I turned to my own mother, an aunt, and friends, (who were mothers), for advice and direction during the first year of Brent's life. My then husband and I were University students on a very tight budget so we were not able to purchase any books on child rearing. However, I did receive, as a gift, a copy of Dr. Spock's <u>Baby and</u>

<u>Child Care</u> book, an excellent reference whenever I needed to understand whether or not I was doing the "right" thing. His advice proved invaluable on those days when I began to panic as to what to do next in caring for Brent.

Brent's development continued to fit within the norm, according to medical professionals and my own comparison of his progress with that of other babies his own age. However, there was one area that was different from the other babies that I observed. I couldn't get him to smile quickly. Yes, he did smile at approximately six weeks of age which was incredible to experience as then I felt he was connecting to the world for the first time in an interactive way. I noticed that other babies his age would smile easily, giggle, coo, and laugh throughout those early months while Brent continued to stare at me with such a serious look on his face. I took up the challenge to see if I could somehow humour him into smiling. These attempts included playing the game "this little piggy went to market, this little piggy went home" with his toes, putting his toes on his nose, and holding him gently in the air. His father also tried these approaches to make him smile. It did not come easily.

We lived in a basement suite near the University campus where I washed our clothes in a wringer washer, then took my baby and the wet clothes in the baby tram to a Laundromat nearby to dry the clothes. During those times, I turned on a transistor radio near the washing machine, propped my baby up in a little chair, and began to sing along with the songs on the radio. I would make funny faces, clap his little hands together, tickle his toes, and tell him stories. Breakthrough — he began to smile, coo, and respond warmly to me. This was very exciting at the time as I was quite worried about how serious he looked at such a young age — only three months old. I had mentioned my concern to the Public Health Nurses and Physicians but they told me not to worry so much. Even though we, as parents, were able to help Brent respond more positively to us and his environment, he always became serious after brief moments of enjoyment, and again, we had to constantly work on humouring him throughout his infancy. This challenge was never lessened; he grew up a serious boy, with sporadic moments of lightheartedness and fun.

As early as seven months old, when Brent was able to sit on his own, he amazed me with his need to organize. Other babies would knock down blocks while Brent would neatly pile them up and get upset if they were knocked down. When he started to crawl he spent considerable time putting objects back in place, and consistently went to our bookshelves and rearranged the books so they were upright and neatly placed on the shelf. As I observed his desire for neatness I purposefully took some of the books off the shelves, left them nearby, and scattered toys in various places. Brent continued to crawl to each area and put everything back in its place, over and over again. He was never content with a mess of any kind, and was determined to keep his tiny world in order. This organizing was done in a serious manner, and only after its completion did he relax and respond to songs, stories, and games with laughter and contentment.

Another behavior that stood out from other children in my extended family was Brent's reluctance to let family members and close friends touch him in any way. Unlike his sister, who was outgoing and friendly towards her relatives, Brent would hang on to me tightly and/or stay close to me during visits and family outings. There was one exception in my extended family—his Aunt Lesley, who never attempted to approach him directly. Rather she would talk to him quietly without trying to pick him up or hug him, and over time, her quiet but warm energy began to bring him closer to her. This closeness lessened my fears about Brent being isolated from my familial network, and I felt very protective towards him when he relied on me to shield him in social situations where he withdrew. I also felt relief when Brent would respond positively to physical contact with his father and sister. Even though he expressed jealousy towards his sister during her infancy, he became quite protective of her in the outside world if he felt she was being threatened in any way.

Most parents, I believe, deal with various challenges in their children's lives, so I accepted Brent's seriousness as my main challenge while he was growing up. He excelled in school, sports, and art endeavors. He interacted and played with his siblings, friends, and cousins in what appeared to me as appropriate for his age at the time.

There was one behavior that became evident during his childhood besides the seriousness of his disposition. Brent would interact with other children who came over to play, and then, ask me quietly to tell them to go home. He often wanted to be alone; yet, when I observed him playing with others he seemed to be involved with them each time. Much of his time alone involved organizing his space although it did not seem overly compulsive to me as he also played with his toys, made figures out of Plastercene, read his books, and drew pictures. I found myself drawing him out of his room, though, as he seemed to stay in there too long at any one point in time. This was not difficult when he was pre-school age, as I would bundle him up along with his younger sister, and take them to the library, tobogganing, skating in the backyard, and visiting my aunt who lived nearby.

Brent was just over two years old when his sister was born, and some of my concerns for him were pushed into the background due to her problems as a newborn. It all started during the trimester of this pregnancy when I developed seizures due to medication I was taking for extreme nausea. I was hospitalized when I was three months pregnant and given other medication to stop the seizures which were very painful, causing partial paralysis in my jaw and neck area. The pregnancy became high-risk for me and I dropped out of University to stabilize my condition at home. My labor was induced two weeks after the due date and our daughter came in to the world close to noon on April 25, 1970. I was absolutely thrilled to have a little girl as I now felt my family was complete. There were no "unusual" comments by the Nurses as her eyes were partly open, and she had no trouble sleeping right after her birth. Problems developed shortly after she came home from the Hospital as we, her parents, noticed she was having muscle spasms when we held her. They were regular spasms, every few minutes, and she was returned to Hospital for observation. Unlike today's Hospital procedures, the regulations did not allow us to stay at the Hospital with her throughout the duration of her stay. It was emotionally painful to see her once a day, after taking a bus to the Hospital and arranging for childcare for Brent, as his father was working at the University. Within a week our daughter was put on a medication, Phenobarbital, for her convulsions, and remained on that medication twice daily for two years. A Neurologist met with us after she returned home and diagnosed her with "cerebral palsy". Immediately I went to the public library and took out several books on the subject as the Neurologist did not give us any useful information, just a probable diagnosis. He told us to go home and wait and see what happens. Fortunately, our daughter's seizures did not reoccur after the medication was discontinued and her parents' fears of "cerebral palsy" or another neurological disease were allayed. Her physical, intellectual, and social development, although somewhat delayed by the medication, continued within the "normal" range laid out in medical charts, and regular checkups with her Physician revealed no further neurological impairments. In my view, her outgoing, sweet, and warm personality helped her brother during their preschool years as she would insist that he interact with her. That insistence often brought him out of his shell, and they would laugh and play together on a regular basis.

During my undergraduate years at University I specialized in Therapeutic Recreation. During a summer job working with children with disabilities, I noticed that some of the children with hearing impairments responded to me in a similar way as Brent did. He sometimes appeared not to understand us, his parents, when we were speaking to him, and at first, we thought he was just being stubborn when he would not follow through with our directions. There appeared to be no signs of hearing impairment during his infancy as he always responded to noises. In fact, he was very sensitive to noises and would often cry and hold his ears when certain sounds bothered him. My observation of the similarity to his responses and those of the children at my summer day camp caused me concern and I took him to our family Physician, only to find out that he was hearing impaired due to crooked Eustachian tubes. This condition was subsequently corrected by surgery but some hearing loss continues to this day. For some reason, I tried to convince myself that my fears of Brent's early behavior were unfounded because it clearly was a physical problem that had been corrected. I was proven wrong. Brent's hearing loss probably did impair his ability to associate and understand concepts during the early stages of his development but the hearing loss was only a partial one and does not explain his unusual alertness right after he was born.

The battle to deal with my fears that our daughter might have undetected neurological damage as well as a growing concern for Brent dominated my thoughts and emotions. Needless to say, the marriage suffered as my husband and I grew more apart — he worked hard on his PhD in Psychology and employment at the University, and I continued part-time studies at the University while raising our two babies. We became so distant from one another that a pattern of two separate lives gradually emerged, resulting in our separation in January, 1973.

Forty years later, as I look back at Brent's early years, and compare his behavior in infancy to symptoms of Bipolar Affective Disorder (manic-depression), it is so clear that these signs were there from birth.

8

The Canadian Mental Health Association, in their guide for families who have a relative with a Mental Illness, **"Who Turned Out the Lights"**, outlines the warning signs of mania and depression.

> *"Warning Signs of Mania" (these symptoms can persist on the average from 1 to 3 months):*
>
> • *Inflated sense of self-importance and self-confidence.*
>
> • *Decreased need for sleep; may only sleep a couple of hours a night.*
>
> • *Jumping from one topic to another and/or talking more and faster than usual.*
>
> • *Racing thoughts occurring almost simultaneously.*
>
> • *Overreacting to stimuli, misinterpreting events and easily distracted.*
>
> • *Excessive social, physical, and mental activities.*
>
> • *Going on buying sprees, being sexually indiscrete, making unwise business investments, or incurring heavy debts.*
>
> • *Having excessive energy, making it difficult to concentrate on a single subject for very long.*
>
> • *Exhibiting moods that affect the person's job performance or relationships with others.*
>
> • *Experiencing rapid, unpredictable emotional changes; happy one minute and angry the next.*

9

- *Refusing treatment because the person may not recognize that he/she is ill.*

- *Blaming others for everything that goes wrong; difficult to reason with.*

- *Losing touch with reality, perhaps hearing voices (hallucinations), or having strange ideas (delusions).*[1]

The trauma of the birth pushed Brent into a manic state that was manifested by his wide-open, bright eyes and inability to sleep. I believe that as early as seven months of age Brent's concern for order in his physical environment was his attempt to control his racing thoughts and internal chaos in his brain. His withdrawal from those around him, and serious expression on his face was the darkness of depression lurking in his mind. Many of the above warning signs became evident as Brent grew older, with the full manifestation of his mania occurring during his teenage years.

Depression was never far behind.

> *"Warning Signs of Depression" (depending on the severity of the depression, the person may experience some or all of the following symptoms):*
>
> - *Changes in appetite and weight*
>
> - *Sleep problems; waking up early, sleeping too little or too much, having difficulty going to sleep*
>
> - *Extreme fatigue; feeling tired all the time, even without having worked, and despite adequate rest*

- *Lack of motivation; procrastination*

- *Decreased effectiveness or productivity*

- *Inability to feel pleasure, "emotional flatness", empty feeling inside"*

- *Either agitation or loss of energy; restless or too tired and weak to do anything*

- *Unusual weeping, sobbing, tearfulness, despairing sadness*

- *Desire for solitude, social withdrawal*

- *Feeling of hopelessness and helplessness*

- *Fearful or anxious*

- *Feelings of self-blame, worthlessness and/or guilt*

- *Fearful or anxious*

- *Difficulty concentrating on work, reading, T.V. or hobbies; "scattered attention"*

- *Difficulty making decisions, even small ones*

- *Recurrent thoughts of death, dying, or committing suicide*

- *Preoccupation with failure(s) and a loss of self-esteem*

- *Non-verifiable physical illness* [1]

Who would have known, back in 1968 that a baby could be born into a manic state followed by ongoing periods of depression that would dominate his internal world and erode his sense of well-being and confidence as he faced the challenges of everyday life. As his mother, I lived with a sense of protectiveness and concern for Brent that permeated all aspects of my life, and yet, I could not explain to myself or others why I felt so affected by his development. I told myself that I was just like any other mother — the sun rises and sets on her children, but I always knew something was wrong. I always knew that Brent was suffering and I was proven right as this devastating disease called Mental Illness took over his life.

2

ONE CANNOT TURN BACK THE HANDS OF TIME

I have always been a person who tried hard not to look back on my life and dwell on my mistakes to the point where guilt and disappointment prevented me from moving on. Unfortunately, there is one major mistake that I made which negatively affected the emotional health of my two young children after their father and I separated in 1973. At first, the children stayed in the family home with me and their father rented an apartment close by. There was tension during the separation but as parents we tried hard to make mutual decisions in the best interests of our children, agreeing that we did not want to be together any longer. Visiting arrangements were worked out between us and we continued to go our separate ways, also agreeing that neither of us would move out of the city.

During the first year of our separation the children visited their father together but as time went on their father expressed a strong desire for custody of both children. I did consider his request but could not accept my role as that of a visiting parent. I could not imagine them being away

13

from their mother's daily care and nurturing. However, it also did not seem fair to me that their father be the visiting parent or that we engage in a destructive custody battle in the courts. I was a strong believer that both parents had equal rights to their children, within the marriage and after divorce should it occur. Fathers were rarely awarded custody in the seventies even in situations where the father may have been the more appropriate custodial parent. I did not agree that automatic custody of children should always be awarded to the mother; therefore, I decided to enter into an agreement with the children's father that he obtain custody of Brent, and I obtain custody of our daughter.

As soon as we decided to separate, we told our children separately of our decision. Our daughter was only three years old and didn't seem to understand what was happening. When her father moved out of our home, she helped me pack his belongings as well as other items that he could take to his apartment. Little did I know that allowing her to participate this way encouraged her, during her childhood, to nurture and care for her father when he was ill, preventing her from experiencing a "childhood" free of anxiety and worry for her father. It is no wonder that our daughter became the "adult" Caregiver towards her father during her weekly visits. She grew up with the burden of that responsibility, when she should have been free to "just be a kid". I certainly was aware of her stress and anxiety when her father was ill but I did not realize that she felt responsible for trying to make him get better each time. I misinterpreted her actions as a child's love for her father and I actually encouraged her in her care giving role. After all, shouldn't a little girl be encouraged to nurture during her childhood so that when she grows up she will know how to nurture her own family? Many years later, our daughter struggled to regain her own identity instead of giving it up by "enabling" others in her personal life. Her journey has taken a positive turn over the last few years and we have been able to stay close and connected, mainly due to her insightful and forgiving nature.

Brent's reaction to the news of our separation was very disturbing. He was told this news in our car, and as soon as we got home, he crawled under the kitchen table and would not come out. I tried to coax him out but he curled up in a little ball and wouldn't move. He didn't speak; just cried and withdrew. I bought him a blanket and some toys but he still wouldn't relate to me. Sammy, his Siamese cat, moved in and out, rubbing against his arms, meowing loudly. Brent was very attached to Sammy and began to respond warmly towards him. Finally, Brent crawled out and went to his room. He was silent for several days after that—just staring and not relating. Slowly, but surely, as I encouraged him to talk to me, he began to come out of his shell, and resume his normal activities. I thought that the crisis was over and wrongly assumed that he was over the shock of the news. Brent did not want to help his sister pack his father's belongings a few weeks later. He would not let his father touch him and he remained silent and cold towards me throughout that period. I began to think that being separated from his father was the problem and that if he spent more time with him he wouldn't feel rejected. My assumptions in addition to my strong belief that a father has equal rights to his children clouded my judgment and I made the worse decision of my life. This was the decision, agreed to by their natural father, to split up the two children; our daughter would live me and Brent would live with his father. We proceeded to file for divorce and attended the court hearing together. We even went out for dinner right after the court hearing, reinforcing our decision to live close together and continue regular visits with our children.

I cannot begin to describe how much it hurt me to pack Brent's belongings and move him in with his father. Each time I felt overwhelmed with sadness and grief, I told myself I had no right to feel this way, that I was being selfish. A boy needs his father; a girl needs her mother. That is the nature of things. This view of the world caused irreparable damage, in my view, to both my children. I was so preoccupied with "feminist" and "humanist" principles in my life that I could not see how much pain my own children were experiencing. I learned of their pain over the years as Brent's Mental Illness came out of hiding, and our daughter struggled with her relationships.

It is not my intent to proclaim that children must always be together with one parent or the other after a marriage ends in divorce. All I know is that my children were close to each other when they were very young, that they played and argued as siblings do, and that separating them should never have happened.

When one makes a terrible mistake, a life time can be spent blaming oneself to the point of self-hate and disrespect. Both my children, through their kind and generous natures have forgiven their father and me for this mistake. The gap in their relationship has been narrowed, and I can see that they care very much for one another, in spite of different values and goals in life. My sadness and regret is still with me. I hope, someday, to make peace with myself.

1975 was the year of even more change after my children's father and I agreed that we would both move to B.C. and live no more than two hours drive from each other. We both decided to start our new lives in B.C. as I wanted to be closer to my two sisters who lived in the Lower Mainland of B.C. and the children's father purchased a farm on Vancouver Island. I was emotionally exhausted and full of regret for separating my children. I required hospitalization and medical care to regain control of my life. During that period my sisters cared for our daughter while I recovered from my breakdown and gained employment. I focused my energy on rebuilding my life, and arranging with my children's father, to bring the children back and forth for visits on the B.C. ferries. Fortunately, their father decided to sell his farm, and relocate to Vancouver only a year after he bought the farm, so once again, I had more visits with Brent, and he with his daughter. One day, their father came to me and asked me if I would take Brent temporarily as he was moving to Vancouver and didn't have a place yet for both of them to live.

That was my window of opportunity! I quickly agreed to this "temporary" arrangement and then proceeded to focus solely on providing for my children, and rebuilding our lives together. The landlord of the house I was renting allowed me to paint the rooms, and I took up the challenge to create a warm, cozy environment for my children. Brent's cat, Sammy, had died in Alberta and Brent was grief stricken when that happened. Now was the time to find kittens for both children and I did just that. On October 25, 1975, my 28th birthday, battling a major wind and rainstorm, I drove with my children to a farmhouse in Surrey, B.C. where they each picked out a kitten. That was the day I vowed to myself that my children would stay together, no matter what. That determination gave me re-newed energy to create as normal a family environment as possible. Of course, I did not know then of sometime in the future when my children would, again, face separation, due that time to their father's emotional illness.

My employment during the next two years involved acting as the Assistant Coordinator in B.C. of Canada World Youth (Jeunesse Canada Monde), a youth exchange program between Canada and other developing nations. Although my office was located in Vancouver, I frequently traveled a few days at a time to meetings in Toronto and Montreal. My children's father was very supportive and took responsibility for their care when I had to go away on business. This was a period of stability; with few argu-ments between us, and mutual respect for one another. However, one event comes to mind in Brent's life that, at the time, seemed a very positive one. Brent was quite adept at making figurines out of Plastercene and began to mold a Christmas scene of Santa Claus and his reindeers. He had decided, at the age of 8, to give this scene to his father for Christmas. I provided a large board for him to work on, and he began his project in mid-December that year. During the four days that Brent worked on this pro-ject he hardly ate or slept. He was wide awake day and night, and even though he would fall asleep at his regular bedtime, within a few hours he was out of bed and back to the "drawing board". I took two days off work and let Brent stay home from school to finish his project. He would spend hours redoing his figurines until every detail met his satisfaction. Even when I thought the project was finished he was not satisfied, and insisted on reshaping each character's features. Finally, after four days, he completed his work, placed it under our Christmas tree, and gave it to his father on Christmas Eve.

During the period between Christmas and New Years Brent became withdrawn and uncommunicative. I thought he was exhausted from lack of sleep and did not realize that these were the early signs of a manic-depressive episode. I also didn't know that his inability to sleep was unusual as I was focused on his excitement and passion for the project. After the Christmas break Brent came out of his shell, ate and slept on a regular basis, and along with his sister, returned to school.

During my employment with Canada World Youth, I included my children in many of the cultural events that visiting youth participants from countries such as Malaysia, Indonesia, and Guatemala amongst others, organized for the Canadian youth teams. However, when the traveling increased to the point where I had be away from home more often I began to feel torn between my family responsibilities and my career. Just under two years in to the job I was given a two week assignment to assist in organizing a youth exchange in Winnipeg, Manitoba. My children would stay at home during this time and their father agreed to move in to my place while I was gone. Two days after I arrived in Winnipeg I spoke to our daughter on the phone and she started to cry. She had misunderstood me when I told her I would be away for two weeks; she thought I had said "two sleeps". That was a very long two weeks for me after that phone call and I decided to resign my position when I returned home. It was not an easy decision to make as the work was challenging and the income allowed me to support my family. It did not feel right to be away from them anymore so I completed my assignments in the office, gave notice to my landlord, and moved my family out to the country. Their father supported this move as he would be less than an hour's drive to see his children.

January, 1977, a rented double-wide trailer and five acres of land became our new home in Mission, B.C. I added two puppies and rabbits to our pet household and proceeded to look for work in the area. Fortunately, I acquired a position as Executive Director of Mission Community Services and we settled down to life in the country. The landlord gave me permission to plant a garden near the trailer and I arranged for after-school care with a neighbour nearby.

Four years had passed since my marriage had come to an end. My children had been moved to different schools and places to live, never having the opportunity to settle down in one place and develop friendships with other children. Although their father and I remained civil and courteous to each other most of the time, there were, nevertheless, heated arguments and disagreements over issues of child support, different parenting styles, and judgments about each other's new lifestyles. The first few years of my children's lives, before the divorce, however, were occupied by two loving parents who tried in our own way to give them a stable home and loving environment, with lots of attention and affection. There were no parenting courses at that time; no "coming apart sanely" counseling available for adults or divorce counseling for children. We were married too young (18 and 20), with little awareness of our own values and how our difference in values would destroy any bond that we felt at the beginning of our relationship. I was barely an adult when my children were born and continued to grow in a different direction from that of my husband. Sadly, we were not alone as many others of that generation went down the same path. Divorce, which was almost unheard of while I was growing up, became more commonplace during the seventies, with an increasing number of divorces ever since.

Brent's reaction to the divorce was not one, single reaction. He relived his pain over and over again through his silence and detachment from those around him. During the two years that he was separated from me and his sister, except for regular visits, it was difficult to get him to talk, smile, and interact in a positive way with others. I tried to humour him just as I used to when he was an infant but he would only move away from me and play with toy soldiers. It worried his father and I when he created battle scenes with Plastercene molded into drops of blood. He spent countless hours by himself enacting wars with toy soldiers and swords which may have, on the surface, seemed a normal activity for a little boy. However, it was the obsession with the drops of blood that disturbed me, and I did my best to distract him from his toy soldiers with other activities.

In retrospect, I now see that mania was knocking at the door and manifesting itself through his obsessive behavior. It heightened the anger, loneliness, and despair he kept feeling as he moved back and forth between his two parents. On a more positive note, I am grateful that Brent has not acted violently towards others during his childhood and adult years, even when his mania has temporarily made him distrustful and paranoid. I am so thankful that he is a kind and gentle man to this very day.

One cannot turn back the hands of time. One cannot relive their life before the mistakes, see those mistakes coming, and head them off at the pass. Regret does not slip away while the clock is ticking. Regret, guilt, and a strong desire to rebuild my family dominated my emotions for many more years to come. Thanks to psycho-therapy during my hospitalization in 1975, I learned how to face my own struggles that were preventing me from acting always in the best interests of my children.

While I was in Hospital during the spring of that year, I experienced for the first time in my life the blooming of the cherry trees in the courtyard. As I walked along the path there with Linda, my dear friend from Graduate School in Alberta, we were awestruck by the beauty of the pink blossoms, as Albertans were still dealing with snow on the ground. That was a defining moment for me: I knew I was ready to start my new life as a responsible single parent, and I could hardly wait to get going. To this day, those pink cherry blossoms every spring remind me of how much I appreciated the support of caring, medical professionals as they helped me deal with my own childhood issues, and gently guided me through a process of self-awareness and renewal.

3

A NEW FAMILY

The countryside in Mission brought a new calmness to my life that I had not felt for some time. It was quiet and serene, and I quickly organized my living space to accommodate our ever-growing "pet" family. My children were enrolled in a country school nearby and I drove to work in Mission on the back roads during the week. They made new friends in school and visited their father most weekends in Vancouver. I had renewed a friendship with Sherry, an old friend from high school and during a visit to her place in Langley she encouraged me to meet one of her friends, Bob, who had been recently separated. My friend had concluded that Bob and I had similar values; that we would be right for each other. I was not interested in meeting any man who was coming out of his marriage, as I had been briefly involved in Alberta with a man who was married at the time. The end of that relationship was too painful and I didn't want to go through that again. Sherry kept insisting that this situation was different but I declined her invitation to meet him. My life was finally settling down;

my children were both with me, and my relationship with their natural father was an amiable one.

My friend did not give up. One day she invited me for lunch, and without my knowing, she also invited Bob to meet me. There he was sitting at her kitchen table, and needless to say, I was quite annoyed with her. His four year old son was playing close by, and I must admit, I was impressed with the positive attention that he gave to his son. The lunch seemed to go on forever, and I remember feeling frustrated at my own attraction for this man. After lunch, he drove me to an auto-repair shop where I picked up my car to return home. During that encounter, I told myself that even though he was attractive and interested in me, I was just fine on my own with my family. No more men for me thank you!

Two weeks later we went on our first date, and as so many others have said, "the rest is history". Our values were compatible — we agreed on the necessity of protecting our environment, raising children in a non-punitive way, keeping an open door for our families, valuing diversity in society, workers' rights in the workplace, and equal rights for all people. We were naïve at the time about the difficulty in joining two families, especially as my new partner was in the middle of a custody battle with his wife.

The first year of our relationship was very intense. We had a strong desire to be together; at the same time we were challenged by the conflict that arose daily between us and his children's mother. In retrospect, I realize that moving in with Bob and his two children during that custody dispute was a mistake as my being their stepmother added to the tension between Bob and his wife. The children were caught in the "crossfire", and, suffered not only because of their parents' separation, but sometimes as witnesses to their parents' arguments while their parents prepared, through their lawyers, for the custody hearing. Right from the start of this new relationship I knew that my role as stepmother would not give me the right to make decisions regarding Bob's children. When I first met I felt compassion and warmth for them as I could see how much they were hurting as a result of the separation. However, it was a relief to see our four children get along so well. Bob's son was 4 years old, his daughter 6. My daughter was 6, my son 8. The children were living with their father when I met him and their mother visited them twice each week. After two years of separation the custody hearing was held. Bob was awarded full custody of both of his children and their mother was granted liberal access.

Throughout the years, my stepchildren sometimes lived with their mother, and sometimes with us. They became older siblings to a younger sister who lived with her parents in Langley, British Columbia (B.C.). Visits back and forth were frequent as we lived near my stepchildren's mother and her new family. We developed a routine of dropping off and picking up our children so that all four children would not be deprived of seeing their other parents. The animosity between us during the first two years, exacerbated by the adversarial court system, was lessened as time went on, replaced by mutual respect and understanding.

Brent seemed to adapt to this new family as he interacted and played with his step-siblings. He was four years older than the youngest but included him in his play activities right from the time he met him. The two little girls became instant friends as well; our three dogs got along, the cats lived alongside the dogs, and we worked hard to provide a sense of stability in our home.

Bob and I joined an "intentional community", moving onto a communal farm in Aldergrove, B.C. from 1978 to 1981. Throughout those years I worked as a Social Worker and my husband worked on a recycling project while managing the day to day operations of the farm. We lived with many different people, raising chickens, goats, pigs, organic vegetables for our farm and a community of people in Vancouver. Community Alternatives Society, a non-profit organization, had received a co-op housing subsidized mortgage from the Canadian Central Mortgage and Housing Corporation to build a low-rise apartment complex in Vancouver where residents lived together in suites. The membership in the city and on the farm partially shared income in order to maintain both residences, fund environmental/ social action projects, and assist lower-income residents with their living costs. The community was committed to growing food organically, thus providing its members with produce, meat, and chicken free of pesticides, anti-biotic, and growth hormones. It was an exciting time of our lives, and our children were able to play creatively on ten acres of land.

Brent enjoyed singing so I took him to an audition in a nearby community, Abbotsford, for the musical, Oliver Twist. He was ten years old at the time. I tried out for the chorus; he tried out for the boys' gang. We were both accepted and began eight months of rehearsals twice a week. The director of the play wrote a part for our daughter in the street scenes as I was always bringing her to rehearsals with us. My stepchildren were living with their mother at this time. It was an enjoyable time of our lives for the three of us; we would come home from rehearsals singing in the car and practicing our lines in preparation for the eight performances successfully held the following spring. Brent appeared to be more outgoing and happier during this period, making friends with some of the other children in the boys' gang. I admired his drive and focus as he applied himself to this project. He also practiced the piano diligently in preparation for lessons, completing several grades before his interest turned to sports. I was beginning to relax and feel less worried about his serious manner, until we were, again, faced with another crisis.

During this period on the farm, both of my children had expressed an interest in living with their father for a year, and although I did not want this to happen, their father expressed a strong interest as well. They moved to his place in Surrey, enrolled in school there, and I became the visiting parent. Not long after they started school that fall I noticed that our daughter was becoming reluctant to return to her father's after her weekend visits with me. I questioned her about this reluctance and discovered that there was no after school care arranged for my children by their father. Our daughter was 7 years old, Brent was 9, and they were left on their own after school until their father came home from work at supper time. As a result of this freedom, our daughter was knocking on neighbours' doors, looking for company, and Brent was doing what he wanted with no supervision. I brought up my concerns with their father but he thought they were old enough to be on their own for a few hours after school. I did not agree and insisted that the children return to the farm with me. Fortunately, there was little resistance from their father and they moved back to live with Bob and I.

There were signs at that time that their natural father was having difficulties in his relationship with his fiancée. He seemed despondent, pre-occupied, and vulnerable. I became more protective of my children during their weekend visits to his place, and one weekend, brought them home early when I found out they were on their own most of the time there. Our daughter told me on the phone that they were alone late one Saturday night, and she wanted to come home. My fears were not unfounded; mid-December, 1980, I came home with our daughter after Christmas shopping only to find that her father had come to our farm and picked up Brent. He told Bob that he had permission from me to do so and that I had agreed that Brent could live with him again. I was horrified; something in me knew that Brent could be in grave danger. Without thinking things through carefully, I left our daughter with Bob and drove over to her father's house.

In my mind, there was no doubt that her father was having an emotional breakdown. He wouldn't let me take Brent home. He told both of us that Brent's father had died on the Port Mann Bridge. Brent and I sat on the couch together and I knew at that point that I had to concentrate on getting Brent out of there safely. My attempts to reason with his father failed as he was clearly detached from reality so when his father ran in to the bedroom, looking for something under his bed, I yelled at Brent to run outside to my car. I raced after him, and frantically peeled out of the driveway as his father came after us, yelling at me to stop. We got out of there safely but Brent was sobbing and very much afraid. Driving back to the farm, I was very concerned that the safety of my entire family could be at risk as I was reminded of a previous, unsettling experience with Brent's father shortly after our separation in 1973. At that time he had shown similar behavior but was not detached from his own person. He had appeared very disoriented and worried about his children so I spent more time with him then to reassure him that his children were still very much in his life.

Brent's father had recovered from that first episode such that I agreed to the split custody arrangement a year later. This time, however, it was much more serious. I was unable to reassure him that he would continue to see Brent if I took him home. The breakdown occurred shortly after his fiancée broke off their engagement which explained the signs of his vulnerability that I had noticed earlier in the year. Therefore, to keep our children safe, Bob and I decided to pack necessary clothing and other items and took all four children in to the community residence in Vancouver where we stayed for two weeks. Members of our community assisted us in running the farm during that time, and shared their accommodations with us in the city. The children missed a few days of school as we tried to assess when it would be safe to return. I had filed a report with the police but there was little that they could offer us by way of protection. There had been no immediate threats on our safety, but I believed that we were not safe until Brent's father regained his sense of self. I contacted Brent's paternal grandparents in Ontario and they flew out to assist their son by moving in with him for the rest of the month. By Christmas Day he appeared to be recovering as well and expressed remorse towards me and his children for what had happened earlier that month. However, I was beginning to trust my intuition more and sensed that my children might not be safe once their grandparents returned to Ontario. They were keeping a 24 hour watch on their son, and I sensed that he was compliant more for that reason, rather than showing a quick recovery. Boxing Day, during a visit with my children at their father's place, their grandparents proposed that the children move to Ontario and stay with them for the duration of the school year. Their father did not want them with me and showed great distrust towards me; yet, he trusted his parents to care for our children while he recovered.

Once again I was faced with being separated from my children but this time it was different. I believed that their life was in danger if they remained at the farm; I did not feel I could protect them from their father, and their grandparents seemed willing and ready to care for them while their father recovered from his breakdown. I let them go to Ontario with their grandparents, although our daughter came home a month later and saw her father with me on supervised visits for another three months.

I spoke to Brent regularly on the phone and visited him several times during the six months he lived in Ontario. Each time I visited I became more concerned at how cold and angry he was towards me. He did not want to come home. He was excelling in school, playing basketball and baseball, and receiving care and love from his grandparents. I felt like Brent was slipping away from me, and when his grandmother proposed to me that he stay another year, I did not agree. For some reason, although he was achieving on the outside, I still believed that he needed his mother to guide him through his childhood and the rest of his family to interact with him during his growing years. His father had also stabilized, and Brent being separated any longer without both his parents did not seem right. I insisted that he return home at the end of June and that is what happened. His grandparents brought him back by train and I remember the tremendous sense of relief when he stepped off that train and walked towards me in the station. I have never regretted sending my children to Ontario for that brief period of time as painful as it was for all of us. I am thankful that their grandparents so graciously cared for them, giving their own son peace of mind as he worked on his recovery.

In the middle of all this turmoil I continued to work as a Social Worker, co-founded the Langley/Aldergrove Association for Nuclear Disarmament, became an activist in my Union, and assisted Bob in the running of our farm. Somehow, I was able to focus on each task at hand and push aside the emotions I was feeling at any given point in time. I would concentrate on my work, organizing peace rallies and vigils, attending Union meetings and events, and engaging in the day-to-day responsibilities of running a farm and raising children, always conscious of my heart racing, stomach turning or anxiety building as I dealt with each crisis in our lives. Needless to say, it was a juggling act at the best of times but after my children returned home from Ontario I found it more difficult to "bounce back" from that disruption in our lives. I felt over-programmed and exhausted from the stress and activities in my life.

There was no doubt that I loved that intentional community — its goals and objectives. I was part of the peace movement, the Union movement, and trying to make the world a better place. However, the yearning for a quieter, less hectic life with my children close to me became stronger. In the past I had benefited from counseling and I turned to counseling again. I knew I had to make changes in my life; something had to go and it certainly wasn't my kind, supportive partner or any of our children.

Counseling helped me address an issue I have always struggled with my entire life, and still continue to struggle with to this day. "Saving the World" and everyone in it has been my "raison d'être" since I can remember. As a little girl I would visit people in Hospital to keep them company and seniors in their homes so they wouldn't feel as lonely. I brought home stray dogs, worried about children starving in other parts of the world, tried to end racism in high school and stood up for friends who were being criticized by others. I was called a "do-gooder", yet, I never felt I was doing "enough good". This sense of duty and obligation to the world has always been part of my psyche so it was only natural to get involved in an intentional community, stand up for workers' rights in the workplace, and march for peace.

Bob and I included our children in many of these activities when they were "kid friendly", as we believed that exposing them to our values would assist them in understanding how important it was to preserve and protect this planet. However, I started to feel that my over-commitment to the "outside world" was taking me away from my family to the detriment of my family. The decision to leave the intentional community in late 1981 was a mutual decision between Bob and I and we relocated nearby, in the same rural area by the end of that year. I grieved the loss of my community for several months as building an intentional community had been a dream of mine for many years. I just could not handle the responsibilities of this commitment (many were self-induced responsibilities), my employment, and crises in my personal life each time they appeared.

How did my children react to this move? They seemed more content in some ways. They both had their own room in the house we rented and less people to relate to on a daily basis. Our daughter told me several years later that she felt she had to share me with too many people, yet, she seemed to relate so well to everyone we lived with on the farm. Brent also interacted in a positive way with other residents but when we moved out he seemed happier with his own space.

Life as a nuclear, blended family was short-lived (three months only) as my sister, her ten year old daughter, and five week old son, arrived from Yellowknife, N.W.T. to visit us in early 1982. Her husband was employed in a lead-zinc mine near the North Pole, and could only visit his family every six to eight weeks. After visiting us in a much warmer climate and our family embracing her family with open arms, the four adults decided to live together with all our children as an extended family. This arrangement would give my sister assistance in raising her children and support for her while her husband was working so far away. Bob and I were impressed with our own children as they accepted their cousins into their lives, rather than

show any resentment toward them. We eventually purchased a home on an acre of land with enough bedrooms
and living space for the ten of us.

Several years went by and Brent appeared to be ad-
justing to our extended family with interest and enthusiasm. He made a hockey puck out of socks and showed his
youngest cousin (who was still in diapers), how to play
hockey on our deck. He would help the baby line up plastic bowling pins and taught him how to throw the ball at
the pins. My stepson also joined in and much time was
spent helping the baby learn how to play active "sports".
My sister's daughter had the sweetest disposition towards
her cousins and played quite an active role in caring for
her baby brother. Although my stepchildren were living
at their mother's home during those years, they usually
visited us mid-week and on weekends. My mother-in-law
moved in with us for two years and seemed to enjoy being
around her grandchildren. She was loving and kind to her
grandchildren who used to visit her and their grandfather
for Sunday dinners in the earlier years. "Grand mere's" de-
clining health led to her move to an extended care facility
in Langley. We visited her often and brought her home to
dinner on a regular basis until she passed away in 1991.

My sister and her family eventually moved back to
Alberta, closer to her husband's family and Bob and I
moved with our children off the acre and into the City of
Langley. Once again, we lived as a nuclear family except
for a six month period when a friend of mine stayed with
us until she found employment.

After my father died in 1994, Bob and I agreed to buy
another home with my sister and her husband that would

be large enough to accommodate six of us, as well as our mother, should she decide to leave her home in Chase, B.C. and move closer to her daughters. Two of our children were married and my stepson was living by himself at that time. We stayed in the Langley area, closer to the free-way, which shortened my commute to work. My mother did come to live with us for two years, moved out when she remarried, and returned to our home in 2003 when her husband's medical condition required extended care. She visited her husband faithfully there three times every week until he passed away.

As I reflect back on those years I am still amazed at how all the children adapted to the various changes in living arrangements with both sets of parents. It wasn't always easy for them, living with friends and family members as they were growing up. However, they impressed me with their willingness to connect to those who lived under the same roof with us. The open door policy that Bob and I agreed to when we first met had, indeed, been implemented over and over again as we welcomed friends and family into our home. We still live this way today.

4

THE MONSTER WITHIN

Mental Illness lurked in the background during the early years of Brent's life in terms of his adjustment to school, family, friends, and extracurricular activities. With each crisis in our lives he appeared to "bounce back", no matter where he lived or what schools he attended. As he will explain in a later chapter, the highs and lows of his mood swings were very much a part of his inner life, and even though I sensed something was wrong, he lived with his fears and doubts every day. He has told me that the years between eight and fifteen were the best years of his life as he felt he was able to control his moods while continuing to achieve in school and sports. He won several athletic and academic awards, enjoying his competitive nature in baseball and bowling. However, his own despair and darkness was heightened at various times and he contemplated suicide while visiting his father one weekend. Brent's sister was seriously affected by that weekend as she was emotionally torn between comforting her father, who didn't know how to handle Brent's despair, and going after her brother when he walked out to his father's barn. She was more than relieved when Brent walked out of the barn and came back into the house.

I was not aware of that incident until several years later and could not stop blaming myself for not knowing what was happening to our children during their visit. Fortunately, Brent decided not to follow through with his suicidal thoughts that day, and tried very hard to bring himself out of his depression. His sister, to this day, still finds it painful to talk about that experience. Over the years I have asked myself so many times: why didn't my children feel they could come to me immediately and let me know what was going on in their lives—their fears, doubts, and insecurities? Is there any way I could have facilitated more open communication with all four children or was I too preoccupied with "making a living", and "saving the world?". There are no simple answers to those questions; hindsight is always 20/20.

Brent calls his mania "the monster", and could not contain it any longer when he entered puberty. Towards the end of his school year in 9th grade we had moved to a new home with my sister's family, and were in the process of building bedrooms in the basement when Brent became overly anxious. At first I thought his anxiety was related to lack of privacy as we had curtains separating sleeping areas during construction. Brent expressed the fear that he had a terminal illness such as cancer and was afraid that he would soon die. One day, as he was crying, he told me that he felt very guilty because he had not written daily in a diary that he had received from his grandfather for Christmas. Bob and I immediately reassured him that he didn't have to write in the diary every day or at all, for that matter. He seemed relieved and gave me the diary to give to someone else. The bedrooms were completed a few weeks later but Brent's anxiety only grew worse. We tried to reassure him each time he expressed growing concern that his body was being crippled by a fatal disease. He was unable to sleep, eat or concentrate on any activity long enough to settle down. Finally, one day in May of that year I received a phone call at work from the School Counselor asking me to pick up Brent as soon as possible. I immediately left my office and drove to the school. Brent was in a high state of anxiety when I brought him home, and thanks to an understanding employer, I was able to stay home for a few days and attend to this crisis.

The High School Counselor gave me the phone number of our local mental health services and I proceeded to set the wheels in motion to reach out for community resources. This was difficult at first as I believed that it was my responsibility to help my children with their problems. I had to admit that Brent was having an emotional breakdown that I could not stop on my own. We attended several sessions with a Psychiatrist in another community as there were no professionals available in our community on such short notice. Brent cooperated by attending these appointments and for a brief period agreed to take anti-depressants. His anxiety was reduced by the medication but he became so drugged that he could barely function. I was not impressed with his Psychiatrist because he spoke to Brent and me in academic language that both of us had a hard time understanding how it was relevant to Brent's distress. After several weeks of heavy sedation Brent told me he didn't want to take the medications and I agreed due to the side effects of the anti-depressants. He received an academic achievement award in Grade 9 but due to his anxiety and depression he was not able to attend the awards ceremony.

Throughout that summer Brent settled down without any further medication but as fall approached he became more and more anxious. He didn't want to return to his high school as he was embarrassed and ashamed by his behavior on the day that he broke down in school. His father offered to enroll Brent in a high school near his place and told him that he could come and live with him as well. After our family meeting Brent appeared more positive and was willing to try a new high school where no-one knew his history. This move was short-lived. He only attended this school for two months as he was uncomfortable with students who were rough and sometimes violent. He asked to return home in November and we agreed that he would enroll in a different high school in our area.

Early symptoms of mental instability were more evident during that year although we didn't know at the time that he was suffering from Mental Illness. When he returned home again Brent insisted on being enrolled in a Special needs class as he was convinced that he was mentally handicapped. The School Counselor agreed to this plan due to Brent's emotional breakdown several months earlier. However, after a few weeks in the Special needs classes the High School Principal and Counselor pointed out to him that he was intellectually capable of entering the regular program. He reluctantly agreed to do just that. These symptoms were manifested in his increasing anxiety over his physical and mental health. He knew something terrible was happening in his brain and he equated it with being mentally handicapped. During his previous sessions with the Psychiatrist the possibility of mood swings as a result of manic-depression were never discussed. The emphasis had been more on situational anxiety due to changes in puberty and delayed reactions to the divorce between his father and myself.

Brent completed Grades 11 and 12 in the next two years and he attended several counseling sessions with a Psychologist arranged by the local mental health services. He appeared to be settling down. He made new friends, excelled in his 10 Pin Bowling League, and had no difficulty being employed in part-time jobs to pay for his extra-curricular activities. I was very touched at the time by Brent's concern for the students in his high school who were mentally handicapped. He interacted with them in the Special Needs classes and showed much compassion towards them. As a result of his concern for their welfare he volunteered to assist them in school as well as organize pool tournaments specifically for them. Brent felt a need to protect them when they were being teased by "bullies" in the schoolyard as he experienced being bullied as well. Brent graduated from High School after twelve years of schooling in spite of the crises he faced during his younger years. I thought the past was behind us. I had heard that teenagers can experience mood swings as they go through puberty and that they usually stabilize when they reach adulthood. I began to relax when Brent spoke about going to College to further his education. He seemed confident and upbeat when he graduated.

As Brent became more stable, I turned more of my attention towards our daughter, who was having difficulty in school. She had lost interest in her academic studies and began to socialize with friends who were, in my view, leading the fast and dangerous lifestyle of drinking, driving, and drugs. I had argued with her for over a year by this time and tried to tightly scrutinize her activities. This was an impossible task as she clearly did not want her mother controlling what she did with her friends. As well, she kept trying to help her father with his difficulties and didn't know how to handle her brother's depression. I made a decision in April, 1984 to resign from my employment as a Social Worker, due to "Social Worker burn out", and as a last ditch effort to change the course of our daughter's life. Brent was doing well in school again, working part-time in a bowling alley and restaurant, and agreed to spend the summer with my brother and his wife in Yellowknife, N.W.T. Although I was home then to put more energy in to my relationship with our daughter I felt that I had to get her away from her own life.

Against the advice of one of my friends, I cashed in my contributions to the pension plan I had paid into while working, and took our daughter to Europe In 1985 for the summer. She was 15 years old and did not want to leave her boyfriend and other friends. She complained on the plane ride and kept checking the time to figure out what her friends might be doing back home; however, our trip to Europe paid off as she gradually began to enjoy the experience of traveling to places she had never seen. I gave her responsibility for our budget on a daily basis as we trekked across England, Holland, France, Germany, Italy,

42

and Spain. We were fortunate to meet friends at various destinations who advised us of the tourist attractions in their areas so that we could experience some of the history and culture. I noticed a significant change in our daughter's attitude after we visited the Anne Frank House in Amsterdam. Anne Frank was the same age as our daughter when she wrote her diary during the two year period that she hid in an attic with her family during World War ll. I purchased the diary for our daughter after our tour of the Anne Frank House and she proceeded to read it with great interest. Her world became larger as she began to absorb the history and consequences of World War ll. When we returned home, she decided to change her lifestyle, finished High School and obtained a University degree in Child and Youth Care. I never regretted cashing in my pension and taking her to Europe that summer, and she has acknowledged that our trip did influence her decision to become a more responsible member of society.

1985 was a good summer. Brent was working part-time in Yellowknife and playing baseball while our daughter and I traveled throughout Europe. I returned home, rested and ready to work again as a Social Worker, although I had to start as an auxiliary employee this time due to my previous resignation. Eventually, I acquired a permanent position and worked as a Social Worker for another four years.

Summer, 1986, after graduation, the signs of the "monster" surfaced again. Bob and I decided to hold a commitment ceremony on the communal farm where we used to live. It was a joyous event where we exchanged our vows followed by a reception where musicians playing classical music for our guests. A few days prior, we had attended Brent's Grade 12 Graduation Ceremony and were delighted with his optimistic view of life. There were no signs of depression or anxiety during that time. Brent amazed us with his physical stamina when he stayed up day and night for almost three days helping us prepare our acre for a volleyball tournament the day after the ceremony. He worked hard on the property with boundless energy, showed no difficulty relating to the people who attended our ceremony, and participated in the sports activities that weekend. I enjoyed his sense of humour and felt he "was on his way."

Later on that summer Brent moved in with his father, worked in various jobs, and assisted his father with his own business. We interacted with Brent on a regular basis and couldn't help but notice his positive, ambitious spirit. He had definitely come out of his depression and was regaining his faith in the future. We didn't know that the "monster" was feeding his renewed energy, pushing him higher and higher into states of near euphoria and intense drive.

I did not see Brent's ambition as a problem at that time. Both his father and I had always been ambitious. We applied ourselves in each endeavor that we undertook, whether it was University studies, employment, or home projects. In my view, Brent came by it naturally, and I assumed that he would go down the same path. After all, he showed a strong need to be independent financially from his parents, to continue his education, and be a productive member of society. He didn't smoke or use drugs or abuse alcohol. Social activities included time with friends he had met in high school and new friends through his Christian network. Although Brent and I didn't see "eye to eye" regarding the application of Christian values, I respected his desire to explore his faith through his daily relationships with others.

The monster of mania can sleep, sometimes for long periods; other times much shorter. In the earlier days of Brent's illness, after puberty, the mania would awaken gradually, thus, making it difficult to notice. It would feed his renewed energy after a dark depression, and gradually take over his mind. His manic behavior was difficult to detect as it was both sneaky and subtle. Months would go by where he was energetic, motivated, and positive about his life. There was no diagnosis at the time from his previous episodes so we continued to believe that he was "just fine".

Worry set in when Brent's drive became more intense—he would sleep less and less, and seemed to talk faster, full of plans and ambitions. Sometimes, his religious ideas would appear fanatical but he became defensive when I mentioned this to him. However, when he enrolled in Bible College to pursue his goal to be a Pastor I supported his plans as he had expressed his desire to follow this career for many years. He did enroll in Bible College, working hard at his studies and participating in social activities on and off campus.

Just when I thought that Brent was on his way to achieving his life goals, the monster took over his mind and drove him in to a high state of energy for several months after his first year in College. He obtained a summer job at a youth centre seven days a week, and drove two hours a day to and from his employment. In addition, he cleaned house for us once a week to earn extra money for College, which gave me the opportunity to stay connected to him. I encouraged him to speak to his employer about reducing his hours of work as he seemed to be overly stressed with little or no time to rest and relax. He was not eating or sleeping properly and could hardly sit still. Towards the end of the summer he would come over to do housecleaning and ask to rest for awhile before he started. He was exhausted and would sleep for several hours at a time, only to get up and almost immediately switch into "high gear".

Several years later Brent told me that a teenager had held a knife to his throat at the Youth Centre and threatened to kill him. Brent had stood there terrified; the teenager dropped the knife and took off. There was no critical incident debriefing and/or post-traumatic stress counseling made available to Brent by his employer. He continued to work there for the summer as if nothing had happened. This incident only added to the stress of long hours at work, commuting too far a distance with little time to rest and relax at home and with friends.

Research on Mental Illness now shows that stress plays a major role in triggering the reoccurrence of episodes. That has certainly proven true in Brent's case. He continued his Bible Studies the second year as the mania had receded, only to be followed by another depressive episode. He was unable to finish this year as he lost his motivation to attend classes, prepare assignments, and study for exams. The Academic load was heavy with little or no room for error. Brent shared his guilt with us when he missed classes and we supported his decisions to withdraw from Bible College in order to reassess where he would go from there. As he was living in the basement suite of his Pastor's home we didn't see him on a daily basis and relied on him to contact us when he wished to visit. He was a young man, making his way in the world but kept in touch when he needed to do so. He decided to look for work and found employment immediately in a bakery close to his residence about the same time that Bob and I went on a trip to visit Bob's extended family in Quebec.

During that visit I tried to reach Brent by phone but he never answered. I felt something was terribly wrong and could hardly wait to get home, only to find him in a withdrawn, uncommunicative state. He was not showing up for work and had isolated himself in his basement suite. This withdrawal was worse than anything I had seen before during his high school years as this time he was barely able to speak. In discussions with his Pastor, Brent agreed to move back home in hopes that our support would help him regain his confidence and positive outlook. This was not an easy decision for him to make as he felt like such a failure to himself, his church, and his family. The Pastor was a kind man who understood depression and encouraged Brent to go back to his family. None of us knew what was happening to Brent's internal thought process; instead, we interpreted his behavior as a reaction to the pressure of academic studies followed by unrealistic expectations thrust on him by his employer at the Youth Centre, not to mention the threat on his life. Perhaps rest and support at home would help him recover and move on.

Brent returned home, only to sink further and further into despair. We became increasingly worried about his ability to function at all, never mind relate to others. He seldom got out of bed to shower, dress, and eat any meals that we cooked. I had never seen him in such a state and I felt helpless in my efforts to relieve him from this depression. At one point, he had not come home for several days and I was frantic in my search for his whereabouts. Family members asked his friends if they had seen him and assisted me by driving around our community to check out places where he had gone to eat out or meet friends. We still did not find him and I became fearful that he had committed suicide as he had told me over and over again that his life wasn't worth living.

During the week of his disappearance I had just started a new career as a Union Representative for a public sector Union in B.C. For many years I had been active in my Union while working as a Social Worker, and obtained full-time employment with my Union in October, 1989. We had reported Brent missing to the RCMP after the 24 hour waiting period and gave them a description of the car he was driving. At work, I concentrated on learning my new job, trying hard to hide my growing fear and anxiety. When I received a phone call at work from the RCMP I started to shake, "my heart was in my throat", and I took in a deep breath. I felt suspended in time as I sat in my office with the door closed. They were calling to request more information about Brent but I could hardly speak. After that call, I informed my supervisor and the rest of the staff of my personal situation. Their empathy and kindness was overwhelming and gave me the courage to keep on working the rest of the week. Brent did return home on his own later that week; he had curled up in the backseat of his car at a rest area off the freeway and laid there for some time. When he showed up at our doorstep we welcomed him with open arms and I knew then that he needed more than our support.

When Brent returned home we encouraged him to seek psychiatric help through our local Mental Health resources but he felt that he was to blame for his lack of motivation and failure to continue his studies. After he returned home from the rest area, he went to bed and slept for two days. We tried to get him up after the first day to no avail so Bob pushed him to get up and shower the second day. I had ordered Chinese food and we waited patiently for him to get out of the shower. It seemed to take forever and when he finally came downstairs in his housecoat he could hardly walk. He sat at the kitchen table, his eyes glassy and vacant, his hand suspended in the air while holding a spoon. He was unable to move or speak. I knew then that he was "shutting down" and needed immediate medical care. We helped him walk outside to the car and drove him to the Hospital, where he was admitted to the Psychiatric Ward.

That was the beginning of our journey through the medical system. At first, in the Psychiatric Ward, Brent refused to take medication but when the Physician explained that he would have to be held down by a Security Officer and given a needle, he decided to cooperate. I had also stood by his bedside and explained to him that the medication would bring him out of his catatonic state. That was a crucial moment for his trust in me was critical; this trust was an essential component in reassuring Brent that I had not abandoned him.

During this hospital stay Brent was given a diagnosis of

Depression by the Psychiatrist on duty. Brent had a frightening experience in the middle of the night during that time when his body went into spasms. One of the medications that he had received was Haldol and he suffered an allergic reaction to that drug. He told me the next day of that experience and referred to one of the Nurses as "an Angel in the Night". She had given him a counter-active medication which stopped the spasms immediately and allowed him to go back to sleep. This incident caused Brent to resist further medications as he remained frightened of possible reactions. He began to "cheek" his medications and only through blood tests were the Nurses able to determine that he wasn't getting what he needed to relieve the depression. It was several weeks of resisting medication before he complied with the Physician's orders. His Hospital stay came to an end three and one half months after he had been admitted.

Life seemed to improve for Brent after he returned home as he talked about plans to find employment and return to College. He became more energetic and discontinued his anti-depressants but I remained concerned as he spoke of achieving goals that appeared unrealistic. One of these goals was his desire to train for the Toronto Blue Jays, a professional baseball team, and when we pointed out to him that, at his age, it was unlikely that would happen he became argumentative and angry towards us.

Brent also started to hang out with a younger teenager, staying out late, and arguing with us when we questioned him about his activities with this new friend. I thought that he was going through a rebellious phase as he had not shown any signs of rebellion when he was a teenager. The friendship continued to occupy most, if not all of Brent's time, which was unusual for Brent who had been a loner most of his life. I had met his friend and did not trust his motives for spending time with Brent. It soon became evident that he was using Brent in order to borrow his car as he did not have a valid driver's license. Brent also shared any money that he had with his friend (his friend did not reciprocate the favour) and he stopped talking about plans to return to College or find employment. Instead, his conversations with us went quickly from one topic to another as he could not focus on any one point. He rambled on and on, arguing with us if we didn't agree with what he had to say. I commented to him how he seemed to be losing weight rapidly as well as not sleeping. After all, a 22 year old man, almost six feet tall should not weigh 127 lbs. These comments only angered him, and I learned that confronting him with his behavior alienated him further from me. I thought I could reason with him when he expressed delusional thoughts only to realize over time that my challenging his ideas was adding "fuel to the fire".

The increased energy, delusional thinking and rebellious behavior came to a head one night when Brent ran up our stairs at 2:00 a.m., made lots of noise in his bedroom, and left the house. I got out of bed and went into his room only to discover boxes of craft materials that I did not recognize. This was disturbing, to say the least, as none of these actions made any sense to me. Waiting for him to return home seemed like an eternity and when he did return several hours later I confronted him about the boxes in his room. Much to my surprise he admitted that his friend and he had broken in to someone's car and stolen their belongings. I was shocked and hurt by his actions as this was so out of character. Without any hesitation, I told him that we needed to put those boxes in my car, go down to the RCMP station and make a statement. He had committed a crime and had a responsibility to himself and society to make restitution. As well, those belongings had to be returned to their rightful owner. Brent did not argue with me and immediately agreed to admit his wrongdoing to the authorities. On the way to the station he expressed his concern, that if they put him in jail, he would not be able to vote for me in the upcoming municipal election. I was running for Councilor and he had helped me distribute leaflets door to door during my campaign. The advance polls were open that day so I drove up to the polling station, Brent ran in and voted for me, and we proceeded to drive to the police station.

In retrospect, I am amazed that he would think of helping me when he was so out of control and facing an interview with the police officer. The Police Officer took his statement as well as the items he had stolen, and Brent was subsequently charged with theft under $1,000. Bob and I never did find out if his friend had been charged with a similar offence.

We went to court with Brent several months later where he pleaded guilty, received a fine, and, fortunately, did not go to jail. After Brent admitted his wrongdoing he settled down and ended his friendship with the teenager. Occasionally he would tell us that he had met him for coffee but nothing else transpired. Many years later Brent and I met this friend who had grown up, straightened out his life, and was working as a Security Officer. Although I was upset at the time with the way his friend used him, I was pleased that his friend was back on the right track. Eventually, I assisted Brent in applying for a pardon after seven years had passed, and it was a relief to him and his family when he received the official pardon from the Federal Government.

This time, the "settling down" was short-lived. Depression was nowhere to be found and the mania came back with a vengeance. Various attempts at employment were unsuccessful as Brent could not suppress the mania on the worksite. He over-socialized with customers at work, engaged in obsessive behavior with non-stop talking, running, and challenging rules and regulations. In the past he had managed his finances quite well but, now, he was spending his paycheque the moment that he received it after he paid us his basic room and board.

Religious fanaticism took over Brent's thoughts as he approached teenagers to preach the Gospel. Some teenagers laughed at him, others walked away. Unfortunately, there were those who punched and kicked him to show their displeasure. We could not curtail his inappropriate social behavior as he would talk to strangers on the street, pretending to speak a language that they couldn't understand. He showed anger towards Bob and when we asked him not to invade people's space. We began to realize that he had little sense of boundaries between himself and others while he was manic, and that he felt he had the right to approach them whenever he decided that they needed to hear his message.

The streets of Vancouver became Brent's new home after he left our home, driven by his high energy and determination to spread the "Word of God" to people who were homeless. I was panic-stricken by his disappearance the first time that he left on the bus as he did not have any money other than his bus fare and $20 that I gave him for food. He filled a packsack with canned goods and miscellaneous items from his bedroom. His room was already full of large items that he brought home in his car. These items included bookshelves, broken down dishwasher, and boxes of stuff that he had picked up in a junkyard. He had hauled them up the stairs on his own one day when we were out and told us later that he was starting his own business selling second hand goods. We could see that the stuff he brought home was not resalable. In his mind, everything was beautiful and held tremendous value. It was just a matter of time before he made millions. He planned to share his fortune with people who lived on the streets, as well as go to other countries to preach the Gospel. We could not reason with him. If we challenged his plans he became hurt and angry and didn't want to see us anymore. My heart felt like it was breaking the day that he got on that bus, mumbling to himself as he took his seat and checking his packsack over and over again. I sat in my car and cried until there were no tears left. There was absolutely nothing I could do; the monster was alive and well, taking over his life and driving him to a place with no sense of boundaries or reason.

I drove home that day and "re-grouped". Whenever I felt that I had no strength left to cope with new developments in the progression of Brent's illness I would sit quietly in a room by myself and pray for strength from God to help me stay focused on the task at hand: finding

Brent and convincing him to return to Hospital. I had no awareness that he was suffering from a Mental Illness as few people in those days spoke of Mental Illness. It was a "hush-hush subject" that brought shame and embarrassment to families when their loved one was diagnosed with this dreadful illness. One of my aunt's, on my father's side, had been diagnosed in her early adult years with a Mental Illness called Schizophrenia, and when I asked my relatives about her condition they did not want to talk about it. I was moved, however, by my uncle's devotion to her all those years; he never gave up on her and tried hard to cope with each reoccurring episode. My uncle's devotion to his wife has influenced me all my life. It has given me renewed inspiration to stay involved no matter what happened along the way.

During the next year, Brent would show up at home and then disappear again. He found his way into the inner city of Vancouver, stopping at emergency shelters for food and rest. I had circulated his picture at the different shelters and filed a missing person's report again with the RCMP and Vancouver City Police. Staff at various shelters would phone me when Brent showed up and Bob and I would then pick him up and convince him to come home. He never stayed long with us and refused to be admitted to Hospital, only to head back to the streets. His belief that he owned his own business was manifested during his time in Vancouver, as he would knock on residents' doors and ask for donations of clothing and other items. Once he had accumulated several items, he would lay them on a blanket outside and try to sell them to people as they passed by. Sometimes he made enough money to buy food and through this activity he would meet people who offered him a place to stay. Bob and I visited Brent at these Christian shelters and even brought a mattress and bedding to him so he wouldn't have to sleep on the floor. The time spent at these shelters would never last long as Brent's mania prevented him from settling down. There were moments when he would acknowledge to us that he should go home and seek medical help but the mania was escalating to the point where he would stop calling us. We found him one day wandering down a street in Vancouver, smiling and singing to himself. When we pulled over to talk to him we noticed that he was not wearing his eye glasses. He had given them to an older man who could not see very well and he felt that this man needed glasses more than himself. We managed to talk him into coming home for a shower and change of clothes, all the time hoping that he would stay at home and let us take him to the Hospital. That was wishful thinking as the mania does not stop and rest; it has to keep going until it burns itself out and the person collapses.

Over the years Brent would tell me how he sometimes hid in wooded areas convinced that he was a warrior fighting against evil. He had amazing physical strength which allowed him to run for miles and miles. When he was younger he was quite adept at track and field and through a local track and field club he competed in several races. He ran like a deer — very graceful with steady, even strides. I used to enjoy watching him compete while marveling at his stamina and determination.

It did not surprise me, therefore, when Brent told me how he ran over a major bridge connecting the Fraser

Valley to the Lower Mainland. Only when he is in a manic state as an adult does he run excessively, often without eating, sleeping or drinking water, even though he is very dehydrated. There was little awareness by him of what was happening to his body when he overdressed during hot weather. Excessive weight gain, followed by dramatic weight losses caused us grave concern for his physical health, not to mention his emotional state of being.

Eventually Brent was admitted to Hospital during a manic episode, after being brought to the Emergency Ward by Police for disturbing the peace. Of course, he did not want to be held against his will as his mania had completely taken over his thought processes. It was necessary for the medical staff to take him, with the assistance of Hospital Security, to "the quiet room" (lock up room) in order to contain his energy. I convinced the staff to let me go in with him to the lock up in an effort to calm him down. There we were the two of us, in a small, bare room with an open urinal and a mattress on the floor. A camera followed our every move as Brent, very agitated and delusional, yelled and pounded at the door to get out. I couldn't believe at first what was happening. I felt like it was a bad dream, something beyond comprehension. On the other hand, I was relieved that Brent was being protected from the outside world and his own irrational behavior. The medication given to him eventually decreased his mania to the point where he fell asleep. I left the room and went home.

During that Hospital stay the Psychiatrist on duty met with Bob and I to give us his diagnosis of Brent's condition: "Brent appears to be mentally ill, and it is probably Bipolar

Affective Disorder". We had never heard of this condition but when the Psychiatrist explained it to us, it all made sense. I actually felt relieved and frightened at the same time. This meant that Brent's condition had no cure, that it probably had a genetic component, and that it is a life-long illness. It also meant, however, that we now knew what we were dealing with and that it wasn't anybody's fault. I will never forget that day; it began to prepare me for what lay ahead. Brent did not want to believe that he was mentally ill and my heart went out to him when he was given the news. He was still very manic, but we managed to convince him to cooperate with his Physician and the Nurses by taking medication designed to subdue the mania. There were times that he refused his medication but soon realized that the more he cooperated, the sooner he would be released. Thus, began his journey down the path of Mental Illness. We had the diagnosis, and I, somehow, felt that it would be easier for all of us because of this.

The diagnosis did not make it easier for Brent, as his condition did not let up over the next twenty years. Yes, we understood the symptoms, but there was no cure. I did feel better equipped emotionally to support him no matter what happened and over time he, too, began to understand and acknowledge that he does have a Mental Illness; that it is probably genetic, as he had witnessed behaviors by his natural father similar to his own.

Life took on a different direction as we moved away from believing that the episodes were solely caused by external pressures and accepted that they were due to a chemical imbalance in the brain. The next twenty years of Brent's life included thirteen admissions to Psychiatric Wards at several Hospitals, where medications were administered to subdue and control the mania. Severe depression followed each manic episode and our Brent isolated himself from friends and family as he withdrew in his own apartment.

Bob and I never gave up on Brent as we accepted that his Mental Illness had become part of our lives and that we would be there for him as long as we lived. That is a "given", and neither of us has moved from that position. He is our son and deserves our love and dedication as he struggles through darkness and despair, trying to make some sense out of his life.

5

STICK HANDLING THE PSYCHIATRIC WARD

Over the last twenty years Brent has been admitted to many different Emergency Wards, sometimes against his will, other times by volunteering to receive medical attention. The Emergency Ward policies were more than frustrating as the long waits (while Bob and I tried to help Brent contain his mania) made it very difficult for all of us. Sometimes he would take off in a manic state after agreeing to come with us to the Hospital. Other times, he would be contained by two Paramedics who were not free to respond to other calls as Hospital Security Personnel were not available to watch him. The last time that Brent was admitted to Hospital in a manic state the Paramedics waited several hours with him, standing beside him to prevent him from running away. There was one Physician on duty throughout the night and the Emergency Ward was full. Nurses were run off their feet and could only attend to the most urgent calls by patients. Bob and I sat up all night, waiting for the "one" Physician to assess Brent's condition. Even after the Physician finally agreed to admit Brent to the Psychiatric Ward, we had to wait for a Hospital bed. It is not only exhausting for family members to wait day and night in the Emergency Ward, but the over-stimulating activities in the Emergency Ward "feeds the mania". On a previous occasion Brent had been taken to an Emergency Ward by the Police because he was disturbing patrons in a pub. In a full-blown state of mania he believed that he was an undercover cop on a mission and tried to resist arrest by the Police when they responded to the pub manager's call for help. Bob and I had been looking for Brent for several hours and were returning from our search in Vancouver when my mother called me on my cell phone. An RCMP officer was at our door at 1:00 a.m. to let us know that they had found Brent and were driving him to the nearest Hospital.

Throughout the night at the Emergency Ward we waited for Brent to see a Physician. His feet were swollen and bleeding from non-stop running for several hours, and he lit a fire in a garbage can in the Hospital washroom to "keep out the demons". In spite of this, we had to argue with the Attending Physician when he expressed his reluctance to admit Brent to the Psychiatric Ward. Fortunately, Brent was given antibiotics to bring down the swelling in his feet, and our fears that some of his toes might be amputated subsided. Brent wheeled around in a wheelchair, laughing and joking about trying out for the Special Olympics and seemed immune to the pain caused by the severe infection in his toes. The next day, when the full-blown mania began to subside he felt excruciating pain in his feet, and I again, pushed for painkillers to give him some relief.

This experience was an uphill battle with the Resident Psychiatrist as she automatically assumed that Brent had gone off his medications because of his manic state. Bob and I advocated for Brent; we were adamant that this time he had stayed on his medications. This Physician was arrogant and rude towards us but we stood our ground and challenged her on the assumptions she was making. Shortly after our meeting with her, Brent was transferred to our local Hospital. It was then determined by medical tests that the medication Brent was taking (Lithium) was no longer effective in treating his mania; that was the reason he became manic even though he had diligently taken his medication every day for some time. We also learned that anti-psychotic medications can sometimes cause long-term damage to the vital organs, and that it was very important that Brent have regular blood tests in order to monitor the level of medications in his body.

That experience left me with a stronger conviction to make sure that Brent would always be treated with dignity and respect by those in the medical profession. I encouraged him to be polite and cooperative, but at the same time, I wanted him to see that just because he was manic or depressed, did not mean that anyone in a position of authority could "talk down" to him and/or treat him in an arrogant and rude manner. As well, I wanted him to feel secure and confident that I would advocate on his behalf when he was unable to do so.

The procedures in most Emergency Wards do not allow for separate assessments and fast-track admission procedures for those persons suffering from Mental Illness. Mania needs to be contained as quickly as possible with medications and appropriate supervision; depression is only heightened by patients left on stretchers in hallways under bright lights. Inadequate staffing contributes to the deterioration of the patients' condition as they wait countless hours for a Physician to assess their condition.

Entering the Psychiatric Ward for the first time to visit Brent more than eighteen years ago was more than difficult — it was confusing and very upsetting, to say the least. One wanders down a long hallway to the double doors, only to step in to a world of rules and regulations, not only for the patients but for the visitors as well. The rules and regulations did not surprise me — the unavailability of any staff to welcome me and explain the correct protocol and procedures did. I was shocked when I discovered that psychiatric patients were staying in the same area as elderly patients. On one occasion while Brent was staying in the Psychiatric Ward an elderly patients had died and had to be removed on a gurney from the ward. Brent was very distressed, along with several other patients at the time.

Psychiatric patients in the ward should not have had death staring them in the face when they are struggling to keep themselves alive. I soon found out from the nursing staff that they, amongst others, had been lobbying the Provincial Government to designate all the beds in the ward for psychiatric patients only, but due to lack of funding in the health care sector this had not been possible. As well, visitors who came to spend time with patients who were elderly were unprepared and often frightened by the behavior of patients with mental health issues. Visitors had to cope with the fears of patients, like Brent, who were convinced that they would die on the ward just like some of the elderly patients had. It took many years of advocacy by community groups, families, and professional staff to achieve funding for a separate Psychiatric Ward, and when it finally was designated as such, the atmosphere changed for the better. Staff, patients, and visitors could then focus on rest and recovery without the disturbing distractions of a mixed ward.

During my first visit I noticed almost immediately that the Psychiatric Ward was short-staffed on a regular basis, as I would visit Brent twice daily in order to reassure him that he was not being abandoned. The Nurses had little time to sit and talk with their patients as they were pre-occupied with administering medications, charting the dispensing of the drugs, and recording behaviors so that the Psychiatrists could review their patients' charts when they came to check their progress. Psychiatrists did not have much time either and I soon realized that the main focus of Brent's treatment was to administer and monitor the medications. Patients interacted with one another which sometimes caused flare-ups and arguments. I also witnessed acts of kindness between them as they kept each other company to pass away the long hours during their stay.

Psychiatric Wards have a life of their own and I spent considerable time trying to figure out how to be part of Brent's treatment plan whenever I went to visit him. Although the goals and objectives outlined by each Hospital that he was admitted to referred to "including families in treatment plans", I did not find that to be so in most of the Psychiatric Wards. Hospitals are institutions with clear lines of authority; visitors come for brief periods of time, and in my experience, are often treated as intruders if they ask questions and express concerns. There is a sense of powerlessness one can feel when Nurses appear annoyed at your questions and/or ignore you as you stand at the nursing station. Seldom did I experience that a Psychiatrist had the time to really listen to my concerns, although over the years, with determination and insistence on my part, I was ignored less and less. The question always came up for me, and still does: "are visitors being ignored because there isn't enough staff to pay attention or are visitors being ignored because the culture of Hospitals only has room for obeying the rules and not questioning them"? I have concluded that as long as visitors of patients who are mentally ill assume they don't have a right to be assertive and ask questions, they will usually be ignored and dismissed by the "institution".

I decided in the earlier years that I did have the right to ask questions and expect answers regarding Brent's treatment and I insisted during each Hospital stay that I was as much a part of his treatment plan as the Nurses' observations and the Physicians' medications. I learned that being aggressive towards staff gets one "no-where" as they quickly "circle the wagons", and exert their authority over you. It is their domain, not that of the visitors, who can be asked at any time to leave the ward. I also acknowledge that most of the staff is compassionate and caring, but that their workload and long shifts take a toll on their sense of well-being and positive contribution to the recovery of their patients. They are frustrated with lack of funding for "quality" mental health in-patient and out-patient programs as well as adequate beds. Patients who are on the road of recovery should not be discharged too early due to a shortage of beds. I can't remember how many times I argued with staff that Brent must not be discharged too early even if his mania had settled as he needed several weeks to regain his self-discipline and rational thoughts. When I discovered that the issue was lack of adequate beds I realized that this was a "political" problem, and not the staff's fault.

Student Nurses were more relaxed and interested in their patients as they were just entering the workforce with ideas and passions, not yet discouraged by the bureaucracy of health care institutions. I noticed that the students were often non-judgmental; that they interacted with Brent and others as adult to adult, rather than in a condescending and patronizing manner. Brent responded positively in his interactions with Student Nurses and allowed them to interview him for their University projects, whereas, he was more guarded and suspicious of nursing staff as he knew they were recording his behavior. The power of the pen is never felt more than in the Psychiatric Ward as the Physicians rely on the recordings of the nursing staff as well as their own interaction with their patients to determine changes in medications. Although I recognized that it was important to observe behavior I also became concerned that a person's behavior will change when they are being watched by someone who has authority over them. How many of us suddenly slow down when we see a police car ahead of us, even if we are not speeding at the time?

It became important for me to stay closely tuned into Brent's behavior as I believed that his behavior was being affected by the Nurses who observed and recorded what he did. In order to understand the "true" nature of his illness I had to separate what behavior was due to the mania and what was artificially created by being certified and contained in the Psychiatric Ward.

There were levels of privileges that the patient had to earn from the day they were admitted. I agreed with these levels as over-stimulation only feeds the mania. For example, it is necessary when Brent is admitted during a manic episode that the staff confines him to the Psychiatric Ward without street clothes and shoes, making it difficult for him to take off without being noticed. In a manic state, he wants to bolt and it is not unusual for patients to run out of the ward and take off into the community. As long as he takes his medications throughout the day and evening, his mania will subside enough so that he can get dressed and earn the privilege of walking out to the lobby, then outside to the foyer, followed by day passes, overnight passes, and eventually discharge. As the mania decreases, Brent's ability to think rationally and follow rules increases to the point where he gains those privileges.

There were times when I would be more assertive with the staff in pushing for privileges, as I felt Brent's morale was negatively affected by withdrawal of all privileges if he disobeyed some of the rules. Staff convinced me that taking Brent out too soon on day passes would over-stimulate his brain and counteract the effect of the anti-psychotic medications. I eventually agreed with them on that point after I had taken him out on passes only to deal with his mania escalating in public places. In spite of the lock-up facilities and other restrictions in the Psychiatric Ward these restrictions did help Brent rest and settle down. Under-stimulation became and still is a critical component to his recovery after an episode of mania.

Psychiatric programs at different Hospitals varied in their policies regarding flexible visiting hours. Several years ago during a manic episode Brent was admitted to a Psychiatric Ward where the policies and procedures re-stricted visitors to the point where patients spent far too many hours sitting around, doing nothing, and waiting for their visitors. Visitors were only allowed to come two hours in the afternoon and two hours in the evening. I soon became frustrated with these restrictions as my office was situated within a ten minute drive to the Hospital, and I was able to visit Brent during my lunch hour. The Nurses, at first, would not make any exceptions to visiting hours when I explained my situation. As well, I often worked late into the evenings so I requested to visit Brent shortly after the supper hour. That request was denied as well. I became quite upset as those visits were very important to Brent' sense of hope and recovery, and after going up the "chain of command" I was able to negotiate more flexible hours. I heard the same frustrations from other visitors and encouraged them to "respectfully" request a meeting with the Hospital Social Worker, Head Nurse, and Psychiatrist, as well as put their request in writing. Too many families felt powerless to put their requests forward and expressed to me that they were afraid that if they complained there would be repercussions, such as more restricted access to their friend and/or family members in the Psychiatric Ward. I could only encourage them to keep trying and was determined to show them that if I could arrange more flexible and frequent contact they could as well. I pointed out to visitors and staff that the loneliness and isolation in the Psychiatric Ward will not help a person's recovery; rather it could counteract the positive aspects of patients receiving medications on a regular basis in a carefully monitored environment. Seldom did I witness disruptive behavior by visitors towards staff that would cause staff to restrict visiting.

Shortly after Brent was discharged from that Hospital, he decided to find an apartment close to his family so that we could provide support when he needed it most. This also meant that when it was necessary for him to be admitted to Hospital we were able to visit him frequently throughout the day and evening. The visiting hours in our local Hospital's Psychiatric Ward started in the morning and went until 8 p.m. in the evening. There were morning support groups and activities that Brent could attend so we usually came to see him after those sessions were finished. Our family took turns visiting throughout the week and Brent's friends escorted him on passes when he was well enough to go out for short breaks.

Many years ago Brent had been admitted to a Psychiatric Ward for severe depression, and was still there on his birthday at that time. Bob, I, and our daughter brought him a birthday cake and presents on that visit. However, he was so depressed he wouldn't accept our gifts. He cried, saying he wasn't worthy of us and wanted us to go home. The cake was shared with others on the Ward and after we sat with him for awhile Bob and our daughter took the gifts home, to be given to Brent at a later date. Brent lay in his bed in the dark and told me to go home, that he didn't deserve a mother like me. He pulled the curtain around his bed so I sat behind it in a chair. I talked to the Nurses on duty and explained that it was critical that I stay with him until his birthday was over as leaving him before that would send a message that I had given up on him. They were quite supportive as I explained that I would sit quietly and not disturb others in the Ward. There I sat, until midnight. Every now and then Brent would move his curtain and see me sitting there, quietly reading the newspaper. I had told him that I loved him, that he was my son no matter what, and there was nowhere else I wanted to be on his birthday. At midnight I asked him if I could say goodbye until the next day and he opened his curtain to receive my hug. That kind of flexibility and support from the Nursing staff was missing in some of the other Psychiatric Wards that Brent had stayed in. That kind of flexibility and support within the system is necessary to ease the pain and suffering of those afflicted with Mental Illness.

I am pleased to say that at the writing of this book our community Hospital continues to offer a flexible visiting program for family and friends and works with patients and their Supporters in determining a treatment plan during patients' stay in the Hospital.

The "push and pull" of tension between Brent, myself and staff has decreased over the years as I became more skilled at asserting my rights and those of Brent, while at the same time acknowledging that the Hospital stay is an important and necessary part of his recovery. I have learned to work with staff and earn their trust. Since Brent lives close to his family in the same community he is able to return to the same Psychiatric Ward each time he has a manic episode or severe depression that he cannot control. Hospital staff, several of whom have been there for many years, cooperate with us and this cooperation makes it easier to focus on Brent's treatment plan.

In terms of medications, I have learned a great deal about the different types of medication for treating Bipolar Affective Disorder and make a point of updating myself on a regular basis. Although Psychiatrists are trained in this area I do not assume that means my own research and opinions are not valid. By visiting Brent every day in the Hospital I am able to discuss with him any side affects he might be having to his medications and relay that information back to the Nursing staff. I learned that the most efficient way to communicate with the Psychiatrist is to prepare written questions which I then give to the nursing staff to put in the Physician's mail slot. I also write down my own observations and requests and ask for a meeting and/or written response from the Psychiatrist. The Nurses do not always know exactly when the Physicians will be making their rounds so I also rely on Brent and other patients to let me know. At first, I was surprised to learn that the Psychiatrists spend little time with their patients and I soon realized that my written questions had to be brief and to the point. As well, when the Psychiatrist speaks to Brent I am often nearby In the Ward and my presence usually means that the Physician will take a few minutes to answer my questions and/or requests that I have put in writing.

The skill of negotiating with the assigned Psychiatrist has been fine-tuned over the years as I usually walk a fine line between staying in the background while Brent presents his own thoughts and requests, and stepping in when I observe that he isn't being heard.

Advocacy played an important role during a depressive episode when Brent pointed out to me one day that it would be easy for him or another patient to jump out the 2nd storey window in the visiting room of the Psychiatric Ward. He showed me how the window could be opened and without bars the fall from the window could lead to serious injury or death. I pointed this out to the Nurses on staff but they said that their own complaints had not led to any action by the Hospital administration. Needless to say, I was very disturbed by this negligence and immediately left a phone message for the Hospital Administrator, followed by an urgent letter which I faxed to his office. In my letter I expressed grave concern for Brent's life and the lives of other patients, and that I couldn't understand how a simple solution to the problem was being ignored. The Hospital Administrator's response was more than timely; the window was secured within 24 hours. One does not always get immediate attention and satisfactory solutions to issues such as lack of funding but it is crucial to never undermine the importance of advocacy when supporting those who suffer from Mental Illness and/or any other type of disability or disease.

Although Brent had managed over the years to avoid the use of alcohol and drugs he turned to street drugs for several months just after he turned 35 years of age. The mixture of street drugs and his medications pushed him into a severe manic state and when he finally agreed to go to the Emergency Ward with Bob and I, we came up against resistance in the Emergency Ward from the medical staff. Brent was completely honest with the Physician on duty as to what he had been taking but to my surprise, the Physician was not willing to admit him to the Hospital. The Physician agreed that Brent should remain in the Emergency Ward for several hours while they monitored the effects of the street drugs, while I argued that Brent was experiencing psychosis and needed to be admitted to the Psychiatric Ward due to his bipolar condition.

The revolving door in and out of Hospital during the next few weeks was not only due to lack of available beds but also due to the Physicians' resistance to certify Brent under the Mental Health Act. The Physician was reluctant to treat his mania unless he stopped using drugs, but I knew that the mania would not listen to anyone even though Brent was feeling shame and guilt for turning to street drugs. My role as advocate came to the forefront as I lobbied and negotiated with the Emergency Ward Physician how critical it was for Brent to be admitted to the Psychiatric Ward at that time. Fortunately, the Physician finally acknowledged that turning to street drugs was not Brent's regular pattern of behavior and agreed with me that Hospital care would decrease the chances of further abuse of drugs while at the same time "put the monster to sleep".

There is no doubt in my mind that this period of hospitalization followed by several weeks in a Boarding Home program gave Brent the time he needed to restore his sense of reason and responsibility. He cooperated fully with the Hospital staff and Boarding Home personnel by taking his medications, avoiding the further use of street drugs, and attending day programs available to him in our community. This experience gave me new insight into the close link between those who suffer from Mental Illness and the use of street drugs to cover up and numb their emotional pain.

Stick handling the Psychiatric Ward policies and procedures is a never ending process to which I play close attention. With every re-admittance to Hospital Brent and I discuss his treatment plan with the Hospital Social Worker, Nursing Staff, and Psychiatrist. I check daily with the Nurses regarding changes in medication and recorded side affects and/or behavior. I reacquaint myself with the language in the Mental Health Act and rules and regulations pertaining to patients' rights, so that I can continue to be an effective advocate on behalf of Brent and others. The sense of powerlessness that I felt the first time that Brent was admitted to Hospital has been greatly diminished as I now view his Hospital stays as another chance to work with the staff on stabilizing his mood swings - mood swings that have become so disruptive to his sense of well-being and purpose in life.

Each of us involved in Brent's treatment program has a significant but equal role. Mutual respect and cooperation amongst the team members can only facilitate a speedier recovery and increase our knowledge, skills, and abilities to provide as much support to those persons experiencing the vulnerability and pain of their illness. It is critical to work as equals with those who constantly deal with their inner conflicts, while at the same time treating them as whole persons. They are not "the mentally ill"; they are persons with a Mental Illness and deserve to be treated with dignity and respect.

I believe that the Emergency and Psychiatric Ward programs are extensions of the community social safety net, and as a Supporter, I have the right and the duty to engage with the staff of these programs in a cooperative, positive manner.

6

BRENT REACHES OUT

From the moment the Psychiatrist made the diagnosis of Bipolar Affective Disorder (manic-depression) I felt relief that we finally knew what was wrong. Until then we were grasping at straws trying to figure out what we could do differently as parents in our interactions with Brent in order to bring the disruptive behavior under control. He had agreed to see a Psychiatrist when he was 15 years old, but, as mentioned earlier, those sessions with the Psychiatrist were of no assistance to him. At the age of 22, after hearing the diagnosis, he still blamed himself for his mood swings and "out of character" behavior and could not accept that he was suffering from a Mental Illness. The Psychiatrist informed us that there was no cure for this disorder and it would be necessary for Brent to take medication on a daily basis, probably for the rest of his life. He also explained that medication to control mood swings was usually administered on a trial and error basis as each individual responded differently to anti-depressants and anti-psychotic drugs. In order to determine the appropriate

dosages and combinations of drugs that wouldn't negatively counteract one other, it was necessary for a person
diagnosed with Manic-Depression to cooperate fully with
their Psychiatrist's prescribed directions. The medications
had to be taken two to three times a day with side affects monitored by the patient, and reported back to the
Psychiatrist at each appointment. It would take Brent more
than a year after the diagnosis to accept that his mania
was not his fault, although to this day he still struggles
with accepting that Depression is also not his fault.

Compliance with medication was not easy as the anti-
psychotic drugs would cause Brent's to shake and his
speech to stutter. Sometimes, when given increased dosages during Hospital stays to bring down the mania, he
was off balance to the point where he would crash into the
walls around him, and lose control of his bladder. Again,
I acted as an advocate, when on one occasion, a Nurse ac-
cused him of faking his lack of balance to get attention,
and questioned my role in challenging the dosage level of
the particular medication he was taking at the time. Brent
was humiliated and ashamed and reached out to me to
stand up for him, as he knew, in spite of his mania, that he
was not acting. I insisted on speaking to the Psychiatrist
on duty and when he reviewed Brent's medical chart and
spoke to both of us, he agreed with me and adjusted the
medication.

Each time that Brent reached out to me for emotional
support and intervention I believed that I was building a
bridge between us and the medical system. I knew that
he would not immediately trust those in position of authority, especially when this authority, from time to time,

was misused. Although, for the most part, the Nurses and Physicians acted in a professional manner, there were enough incidents of misappropriation of authority to re-affirm my belief that the role of advocate for Persons with Mental Illness is an essential component in each rest-and-recovery period after a reoccurrence of the illness. Brent's reaching out and building a trusting relationship with me gave me the opportunity to discuss each incident as they came up, and encourage him to give me the information I needed to fight on his behalf when he was too vulnerable to do so on his own.

During the Hospital stays I observed how often he would reach out to other patients. He showed compassion, humour, and kindness over and over again to many people, even while fighting his own mania and depression. It was not unusual for Brent to organize pool and card games in the Psychiatric Ward. He would collect empty plastic bottles so that the money from these bottles could buy pizza for those who wanted to participate in movie night. If another patient was crying or staring into space, Brent would try to talk to them, ask them if they wanted to go for a walk, play cards, go to the "smoke hole" and/or participate in the arts and crafts room. He would express how sad he felt for those who hardly ever or never received visitors, and comment on how fortunate he was to have parents and other family members visit him. Sometimes he would break the rules by "taking off" with other patients, only to return later on his own or be brought back by a Security Officer. At some point, after he had left the Hospital against the rules, he would try to convince those who had escaped with him that they needed to return to the Hospital where they could continue to receive their treatment, as he became concerned for their safety in public. Friendships were developed in the Hospital, and Brent would ask me on a regular basis where patients could go for housing, food, and other services. It never failed to amaze me how many patients were discharged to little or no resources, only to relapse and end up in Hospital again. Brent felt a deep sense of responsibility for those around him and relied on my knowledge of community resources to help other patients. He would give them phone numbers of shelters, support groups, and crisis lines, as well as addresses of food banks, Salvation Army and Mental Health drop-in centers, and Ministry of Employment and Income Assistance where they could apply for financial assistance. His compassion and concern for others has never lessened over the years in spite of his own pain and suffering.

Concern for others did not end each time that Brent was discharged from Hospital. Just over a year after he accepted that he must take medication on a daily basis, he asked me to help him organize a support group in our community for Persons with Mental Illness. We had attended other support groups organized by the **Mood Disorder Association of British Columbia** which gave Brent the idea to arrange one in our own community. Through our local Mental Health service, he was able to find a meeting room free of charge and we proceeded to make plans for our first meeting. Resources such as guest speakers, videos, and educational materials were provided by the Mood Disorder Association of B.C. Brent applied for and was successful In receiving a government grant that allowed us to buy a TV, VCR, and videos on Mental Illness for the group. My role in the group was to co-facilitate with Brent, as well as provide support to Supporters. Brent shared his experiences and encouraged others to do the same. There were so many stories to tell; so many stories to hear about isolation, shame, and despair. Supporters would phone me when they were desperate to talk to someone who could understand their fears. I encouraged them to come to our group.

We co-facilitated this group for five years in our community, and during that time, I realized that Brent was clearly a leader, shown by his ability to organize events, bring people together, listen to their pain, provide humour and understanding, and educate them on community resources available to them.

In our community, a Mental Health non-profit society, called **Stepping Stones Community Services**, had secured funding to build a facility and provide daily activities, programs, and meals to Persons with Mental Illness. We were able to donate the equipment and videos to that organization and many of the people who had come to our support group continued to participate as members of Stepping Stones. Brent's illness returned with a vengeance as he struggled to hold back the mania and we had to discontinue our involvement as leaders of our local support group.

Fortunately, support groups continue to grow in our province as the Mood Disorder Association of B.C. provides programs and resource persons for these groups. Just as Brent spent five years helping others cope with their illnesses, so do many others (who also suffer from Mental Illness) facilitate self-help groups.

Brent's reaching out had extended beyond our family. He had given five years of his life to helping others while he struggled to reach his own goals. For many years he had refused to apply for income assistance as he was adamant about paying his own way through life. As his parents, Bob and I helped him out financially (when he would accept our help) but I also encouraged him to apply for disability benefits provided by the Provincial Government. He would pay his bills by working at various jobs but could not sustain employment once the mania took over. The medical diagnosis of Manic Depression convinced me that it was appropriate for Brent to receive a disability income, and my knowledge and previous experience as a Social Worker assisted me in providing the support he needed to "get through the system" and apply for benefits. I could not prepare him, however, for the humiliation and shame he felt when he applied for disability benefits, but he accepted my help as I showed him how to apply and appeal a decision if he was turned down for assistance. As always, the bureaucracy took hold, but I managed to convince Brent to persevere. I could not change how he felt, but at least, he could pay his rent, utilities and food with the disability benefits he received on a monthly basis. That is all he could pay as the amount is inadequate to assist anyone to live above the poverty line.

When Brent first received benefits, Persons with Mental Illness were not allowed to work without most of the money they earned being deducted from their disability income. The earned exemption has increased over the years but is still far from adequate for a person with a disability to achieve an adequate standard of living on a combined disability and part-time employment income. Brent has lived in several different places throughout the years as he could not afford the rent in some of these places when the rent was raised by the landlord. He managed his small income as best as he could, but during mania, he would share every last cent with others whom he deemed less fortunate. I used to encourage him to stay home with us to reduce his expenses, but as he got older, he became more determined to be as independent as possible. He has often said to me, "it is important that I have self-respect and dignity and living on my own gives me some of that".

Many years ago I assisted Brent in applying for subsidized housing through our Provincial Housing Program. The waiting list, especially for single persons, was very long — over five years. After seven years I checked in with the Housing Program, only to find out that after five years his file had been closed because he had not put in another application. Needless to say, I was upset, as Brent had not been told that he had to do this and this information was not included in the original application form. As is so often the case, if an advocate does not "push the envelope" for Persons with Mental Illness so that they can receive programs and services of which they are entitled, the bureaucratic system does not respond. Brent had been reluctant to receive services as he wanted to provide for himself in life, so unless I followed up for and/or with him, he continued to be destitute without his parents' assistance. Finally, he agreed that I could set up an appointment with an employee from the BC Housing Program in order to apply again for subsidized housing. He was interviewed and accepted into the program and put on a waiting list

HOPE THROUGH COMPASSION AND DESPAIR

for a bachelor apartment in our community. This waiting list was much shorter, and he was approved to live in a bachelor suite with a rental subsidy. The increased monies available to him means he can pay his utilities, phone, cable, and groceries as well as access a subsidized meal program offered to the residents in the housing complex.

Each time that Brent accepted more assistance such as his disability pension and subsidized housing it reminded him, again, that he was not self-sufficient, gainfully employed in a career that he found challenging and rewarding. Reaching out to these services also increased his awareness that there was some funding for part-time studies at College for persons with disabilities. He had paid off a small student loan that he received during his first year in Bible College, and did not want to borrow additional money for his education. A career in Sports Broadcasting was another option that he had considered and a program was available in a Technical College close to our community. Brent completed his application to the program, wrote and passed a computer exam, and was admitted to full-time studies in the mid 1990's. As well, he received a grant for his first semester tuition due to this disability.

The first two months of College were filled with promise and hope as Brent pursued his studies with diligence, discipline, and passion. He worked hard on his assignments, studied for exams, and enjoyed the company of other students in the broadcasting program. The daily commute from his apartment to the College added over three hours of driving to his day, and by November of that year, he started to show signs of stress and anxiety over the pressure he was feeling with full-time studies and the exhaustion of the commute. He decided to move closer to the campus after Christmas which reduced the time spent in traffic by two-thirds. However, his anxiety increased, and signs of mania started to appear such as sleepless nights, non-stop talking, and lack of concentration on the tasks at hand. Unfortunately, he had to withdraw from College and move from his room and board situation near the campus because the landlord became frightened of his manic behavior. In a hypo-manic state, Brent managed to find another apartment to rent, but was no where to be found on the day he was supposed to move. Members of our family assisted Bob and I with the move, and thanks to an understanding landlord, we were able to obtain a key and set up his apartment for him.

I knew that he was out in the streets somewhere and became very concerned for his safety. He had enjoyed his College program so much and tried very hard to control the mania by taking his medication as prescribed. The stress and pressure of his studies pushed him in to a manic state such that even the prescribed medication at the time could not protect him from losing control. I began to realize that treating Manic Depression did not stop with medication as stress played a major role in triggering a reoccurrence of the disease. I would learn over the years that managing this stress would be a critical component in achieving stability and balance over the longer term.

Brent's subsequent hospitalization and recovery took over two years as severe depression followed the two months of mania. He was devastated that he could not complete his College program. The reoccurrence of mania this time caused so much despair that I became fearful for his life. He had lost faith that he could ever develop a career, become self-sufficient, and eventually get married and have a family. He thought he had the illness under control to the point where it would not take over his life again; this setback brought on a two year depression where he was hardly able to speak, gained excessive weight, and stayed at home with us so we could support him in any way possible.

During this setback reaching out to others included only Bob and I, and we attempted to motivate Brent as much as we could. He agreed to come to movies with me as he would often say that two hours in the movie theatre gave him some relief from his despair. Ever since he was 4 years old I had taken him to Canadian Football League (CFL) games. We both enjoy watching the games and supporting our team, the B.C. Lions. No matter how many days he had been in bed, barely able to get up in his depressive state, he managed to come to the games with me during the CFL season from June to October and watch the semi-finals and Grey Cup on television.

Over the years I recognized that going to a game when Brent is in a manic state only feeds the mania, due to the over stimulation of more than 25,000 fans cheering for their team. However, our season tickets provide a structure where he can momentarily escape a little from the darkness in his life. Also, it never fails to amaze me how he still remembers football statistics from years past and continues to retain current statistics in spite of his inability to communicate in conversation during his depression.

Gradually over the years as Brent began to understand the cycles of his illness, he reached out to other persons suffering from Mental Illness. As mentioned earlier, he had participated in programs offered by a non-profit society, Stepping Stones Community Services, and through these programs began to develop friendships with other members. They played pool and cards, watched movies, went out on field trips, ate meals, and volunteered their services when they were able to do so. I was fortunate to meet his friends when Brent invited them over for dinner on special occasions such as birthdays, thanksgiving, Christmas, and New Years, and was deeply touched by their kindness and support for one another. I became aware of their struggles, their sincere attempts to deal with the stigma of Mental Illness and their ongoing efforts to find meaning in their own lives. They would visit each other when one ended up in Hospital even though being there sometimes triggered their own memories of previous stays in the Psychiatric Ward. They would take each other out on passes to assist in reducing the loneliness often felt when spending weeks, and sometimes months, in treatment. As each one struggled with relapses and setbacks, the others would show empathy and patience, waiting for mania to subside and/or depression to lift. The depth of their friendships has taught me the importance of "being there for one another" during misfortune and tragedy.

As parents, Bob and I have walked a fine line between providing support and taking control of Brent's activities. Through Brent's understanding of his illness over the years he has reached out to us by agreeing to our intervention when necessary. We have his permission to enter his apartment with a set of keys that he has given to us when we haven't heard from him for more than three days, as he realizes too much isolation during a depressive episode will drive him further into despair. During a manic episode he allows us to remove possessions from his apartment and put them in storage as he knows that he would give everything away to others. He trusts us with his disability pension by turning his money over to us so that we can pay his bills for him while he is recovering. We have explained to him that our wills state that any money he might receive would be put in a trusteeship, with his sisters as set guardians of that Trust. He has accepted the importance of protecting his interests in that way. Even when Brent is heading towards full-blown mania, the trust that we have built up over time with him stays intact. This trust is at the core of any support we give to him.

In spring of 2005, Brent turned to gambling for the first time when a local casino was opened in our community. He had turned to street drugs, as mentioned earlier, and reached out to a support group, Narcotics Anonymous, which assisted him in understanding the pitfalls and dangers of drug addiction. After several months of gambling he agreed to allow Bob and I to handle his disability pension so that he would not lose it all in the casino. He expressed to us the guilt and shame he felt when he gambled and wanted to restore his sense of morality and responsibility for his finances. A close friend of his had also turned to gambling and he could see how destructive it was when she was no longer able to pay her rent, buy groceries, and spend time with her friends. The gambling had taken over her life, and when she agreed to go to an addictions counselor with him, and then cancelled, he decided he had to get help for himself. When Brent told me that he had picked up a brochure at the casino and phoned to book an appointment with a Gambling Addictions Counselor I was again touched by his willingness to reach out for help. The appointments took place on a weekly basis and he cooperated fully with his Counselor throughout that period. After three months of my handling his money, and giving it to him three times a week, Brent decided to try and manage it on his own. His urge to gamble had diminished as he applied the knowledge he acquired through his Counselor, and allowed the support from the program to guide him away from the casino life. Brent continues to enlist our support to assist him in managing his finances whenever he feels that his desire to gamble might interfere with his financial responsibilities. At the writing of this book, he has not suffered a relapse by using drugs or engaging in gambling for more than three years.

Both mania and depression make it difficult for Brent to take care of the basic necessities of life when he is experiencing relapses. His reaching out for support from Bob and I allows us to assist with paying his bills, cleaning his apartment, doing his laundry, and going with him to his psychiatric appointments. When he is ready to assume responsibilities for day to day activities we step back until he requests further assistance. Although we have encouraged him to accept our help when needed, we have also been willing to let go of this responsibility as soon as he acquires enough stability to handle his own affairs.

Brent sometimes resists our support as it reduces his independence, but his insight in to his own illness has enabled him to recognize that too much isolation will only cause further deterioration of body, mind, and spirit. The darkness of Depression makes it very hard for him to reach out; that is when we reach out to him. With patience, compassion, and understanding we gently encourage him to let us into his world; he may resist at first, but eventually agrees to accept our support.

7

LETTING GO

As a Supporter, I have learned that there is still not a magic formula, exact dosage of medication or cure for Brent's Mental Illness. I have learned that I can only be involved as long as he allows me to be there for him and with him. Unconditional love for him has always been there, and his acceptance of my participation in his life, as well as others in our family, constantly recharges my emotional battery. He continues to reach out to his family, friends, and community resources even when he isolates himself from the outside world for several days at a time during periods of depression.

Letting go is a process with a beginning but no end. I do not believe that there will ever be a day when I can say that I have finally "let go of the urge to find the cure". However, my energy is now directed towards keeping myself as healthy as possible so I can just "be there for Brent". The holistic approach to health appeals to me more because I believe that it integrates one's body, mind, and spirit. This integration can bring a sense of inner peace and calmness to situations that otherwise may feel stressful and disjointed. It is not easy to focus on myself, especially when my mind and emotions are preoccupied with what might happen next in Brent's life. I can only ignore for so long, however, the arthritic inflammation in my back and shoulders, migraine headaches, and increasing physical and emotional exhaustion. I coped better with these symptoms twenty years ago when we first got the diagnosis of Manic Depression, but the aging process is taking its toll on my body. Therefore, I find it more necessary to take better care of myself as I want to be a support to Brent as long as possible.

Fortunately, I was able to gear down from full time to part time work at age 57, which has allowed me to turn my attention to a healthier lifestyle. Before retiring from my career, the juggling act between work, family and community involvement was a constant challenge and balancing act. When I organized women's conferences on the theme of "Balancing it All" I realized how much women, in general, have to balance in order to fulfill their commitments to work and family. So often we learned at these conferences that we didn't spend enough time taking care of ourselves, and that, without this care, we would end up unable to keep up our commitments. Thus, we shared ideas and stories on how we could better nurture ourselves, recognizing that this nurturing would go a long way to helping others. My work as Education Officer in my Union assisted me in understanding that many other trade Union women face the same struggles that I did on a daily basis. So many of us are coping with parents who are aging and family members and friends who are disabled or ill, all of whom may need our love and support. At the same time we go to work committed to doing our jobs as skillfully and efficiently as possible. I actually met many women who were juggling more critical family situations than my own, and I gained much strength and motivation from their courage and determination. I interacted with these women and learned that their sense of humour, deep sense of compassion for others, and commitment to their employment and families guided them through their darkest days. They were my role models and I became more determined to handle whatever came my way. Always I kept in mind that "there but for the Grace of God go I", as I persisted in maintaining a humble perspective on all that was happening in my life.

For many years, while I was working, there were several co-workers and Union activists who showed compassion during times of crises, especially when Brent was missing or hospitalized. This type of understanding is very important when a Supporter is trying to balance work with family responsibilities. It is difficult to mention everyone as there were so many. However, two individuals stand out: Patrice Pratt, my Direct Supervisor while I was Education Officer, and John Shields, the President of my Union, who touched me with their flexibility and warmth. They never doubted my work and valued it highly as I developed education materials and programs based on "participant-centered learning". John Shields showed kindness, wisdom, and patience. Patrice Pratt, who had raised her daughter born with Williams Syndrome, gave me endless ideas and energy as she showed me how she overcame so many obstacles in the way of her daughter's social and educational development. In my darkest moments Patrice would, and still does, give me unconditional support while at the same time updating me on available resources and programs for people with disabilities.

The Physician's diagnoses of Bipolar Affective Disorder gave me the focus I needed to research and understand as much as I could about Brent's illness. I thought at that time that if I could learn about the symptoms, medications, and treatment available I would then be able to educate Brent and assist him in coming to terms with the illness. As long as I was searching for information I felt, somehow, that I might find a cure out there - some type of therapy, medication, and/or unknown resources that would give me the answer. This search went on for years and each time that I discovered new information I became more hopeful. I tried to pass this hope on to him, especially when he was experiencing the depressive part of the cycle, only to discover that when he is in a state of Depression he closes off the world and everyone in it. My words of encouragement could not reach him during darkness and despair and I began to wonder if these words might have made it worse for him. As I learned more about Depression I realized that phrases such as "things will look better tomorrow" or "you have a lot to live for" may actually do harm to a person who already feels alienated from those around them. I began to struggle with myself, doubting my own optimism, and anxiously rephrasing what I would say to him if he didn't respond. I became silent in Brent's company with very little to say as I began to understand that treating Depression is not as simple as expressing what you might think is supportive and helpful.

Over time I discovered no matter what information I was able to find, Brent continued to go through his cycles of Mania and Depression. The information assisted me in lobbying with Psychiatrists and Nurses in the Psychiatric Wards especially when it came to prescribing different medications and increasing or decreasing dosages. I also attended information sessions on Mental Illness provided by various community resources and became much more aware of the day to day struggles and accomplishments of those who faced great adversity. During these sessions I met dedicated medical and mental health professionals who strive to educate all of us on Mental Illness. The education forums over the years have included more and more testimonials from people with Mental Illness, who through their stories, have helped reduce the stigma of this disease and given others hope that they, too, have the right to be respected and accepted by society.

Brent reminds me from time to time that I have to "let go" of trying to shape the course of events in his life. This reminder gets me back on track to being a supportive parent, rather than a controlling parent. As a mother, it is always easier to revert back to giving advice even when my children don't particularly want to hear that advice.

At some point during this process of "letting go" I realized that the best way in which I could help Brent was to take care of my own health in every aspect. Having suffered from back pain for years and avoiding a spinal fusion due to appropriate back care through fitness and weight reduction, I knew that stress would always go to my back. My back became my ally, in that it would send me early warning signs that I must rest and recover in order to handle the demanding pressures of my work and cope with the cycles of Brent's relapses. I had also gained extra weight over the years while I was traveling on my job, eating in restaurants and at banquets on a regular basis. Spending considerable time in airports, hotels, and on the road made it difficult to focus on healthy eating patterns and regular exercise. The typical ten+ hour work day left little time to fit in any stress reducing activities. It took almost six months of sick leave, flat on my back in excruciating pain for me to finally "wake up and smell the coffee". During that time, as I struggled with the daily tasks of living and managing pain, I realized that I had to take a proactive approach to restoring my health and learning to balance the pressures in my life. I had tried in earlier years to achieve this balance but always managed to get off track as soon as new challenges came my way. This time I knew that I had to stay on track and do everything in my power to become healthy again. How could I visit Brent in the Hospital when I couldn't even move without almost passing out from the pain? In 1986 when I ended up in Hospital with severe back pain and subsequently recovered at home during a four month period I learned to knit lying flat on my back. Fourteen years later, I decided I had to focus on understanding my personality and how I tended to ignore early warning signs, take on more commitments, and disconnect from the physical part of my being. I knew that this was a turning point for me where I would have to shed old habits and learn a different approach to handling responsibilities.

"Balancing It All" did not just involve effective time management but a new way of thinking. I have always been very competitive, mostly with myself, and have not changed that part of my personality. However, I concentrated on getting in touch with the other side of my nature — the need to rest, to read, to learn to be quiet and alone, and re-engage with those activities in my childhood that restored my energy.

Intellectual and academic achievements through work and volunteer activities had to be shared with other pursuits that would help me become a more integrated person. I listed what these activities should be, struggling with an inner voice that said I was being selfish to pursue anything that would bring me a sense of contentment. After all, it was my mission in life to "save the world", "help others", and sacrifice my own personal needs for the common good. Lying flat on my back, depending on my husband to take over all the responsibilities in our lives wasn't exactly helping anyone, including myself.

Fortunately, I was able to secure a transfer closer to home in my employment which ended the long commutes, traveling, and eating-out life style. It did not end working long hours as that is standard for any Union Representative who works for a Union. My new office was so close to home I could drive there in less than five minutes, and I realized that this new lease on life was handing me an opportunity to put into practice all the ideas and plans I had come up with during my convalescence at home.

Little did I know that the increasing demands of the workplace due to a reactionary, right wing government would make it an even greater challenge to achieve the balance that I knew was necessary for me to become a healthier person. During that period thousands of workers lost their employment due to contracting out; others had wages reduced and benefits decreased. Those who hung on to their jobs were expected to "work harder, smarter, faster", putting a tremendous strain on the remaining workforce. Unions fought back and worked in overdrive to fight these changes and lobby community organizations and public citizens to protest these draconian measures. This fight was not in vain as during the next five years through solidarity and collective action, the voters in our province elected many representatives who are more supportive of workers' rights and public services. The struggle never ends, of course, as workers' gains can be lost without political and public support of their issues.

Physical fitness programs, re-engaging with music through joining a choir and community band, taking French courses through Continuing Education Programs, as well as gardening, became my stress relievers as I met the challenges of workload pressures and Brent's manic episodes and subsequent hospitalization. Although I couldn't run due to back problems, I trained for charity walks and enjoy participating in them to this day.

Regular training for these races strengthened my back and the pain was greatly reduced, to the point where I no longer had to take daily medications. As well, the exercise reduced stress on my body that resulted from the long hours on the job. Singing and playing music involves deep breathing and concentration, thus distracting me from negative thought patterns and feelings of hopelessness as I watch Brent go through his mood swings. Taking French courses over the years has and continues to be a passion of mine as I enjoy learning about the French culture in France and Quebec, and feel a sense of accomplishment when I can communicate with others in their own language. Gardening involves the seasons of life, and each season reflects its own beauty and uniqueness in the flowers and vegetables that I grow. Paying attention to the earth through the use of organic materials and fertilizers and nurturing my garden restores my faith, that in some way, we can make a difference if we take care of our environment, our families and our friends.

It was not easy to leave my workplace and retire in December, 2004 without feeling guilty that I was "letting down" the members that I represented over the years. However, the spirit and enthusiasm of the younger generation as they fill Union positions made me realize that Union solidarity is alive and well in the labour movement, and that handing the torch to those coming behind me was necessary for me to "let go" of that part of my life. Of course, I will always be available to assist in election campaigns, rallies, protests, petitions, and vigils that remind us all that "what we desire for ourselves we should desire for others".

For the first time in over 40 years I now have the opportunity to live my life more involved with family and friends, self-development, community volunteer activities, and environmental and social issues. There is more time to reflect and appreciate the moment, to just "be" with Brent" no matter what he is experiencing at the time. I enjoy his company even when he is silent, as his silence is a reminder that I must be patient, kind, and sensitive. His humour keeps me laughing, and his warmth when he is able to relate, touches me always.

Letting go of expectations opens the door to new experiences through an open mind and renewed spirit. It has been my greatest struggle in life and I will probably continue to wrestle with the temptation to "take control" of something. However, I now experience a sense of relief as I realize that not being able to control everything allows me to receive support from others in a gracious and appreciative manner, thus enriching their lives and mine.

8

THE ROLE OF SUPPORTER AS ADVOCATE

The role of Supporter can be difficult, especially when one is emotionally close to someone who struggles with Mental Illness. So much of one's time is taken up by emotional turmoil which may parallel the ups and downs of the person as they go through their manic-depressive cycles. These emotions often prohibit the Supporter from staying objective and neutral, thus blocking the ability of the Supporter to "be there" for their loved one in a positive way.

In previous chapters I have stated how important it is for Supporters to educate and update ourselves on research available on Mental Illness so that we can be better informed on causes, symptoms, and treatments for those suffering from this devastating disease. We can also provide better support by learning how to let go of trying to control the lives of those we want to help, and instead, provide unconditional love and guidance. Although our love and guidance is the key to letting others know that we will not abandon those whose inner world is full of darkness, despair, and confusion, we also need to be the link between them and the outside world. This link can only be established and sustained if we learn to be an advocate in school, community, healthcare, social services and employment programs.

The definition of "Advocate" stated in Webster's Encyclopedia Dictionary, Canadian Edition is as follows:

> *"Advocate—a person who pleads on behalf of another; a person who speaks or writes in support of some cause, argument or proposal. Advocate approach: supportive measure for aiding mental health Patients in dealing with bureaucracy to show that difficulties can be mastered".*[2]

Although this definition does not outline that the Advocate must be "outside of themselves", so to speak, it is clear to me that pleading on behalf of another means speaking for them and/or with them. The focus must be on the task at hand and not serve as an outlet for the advocate to talk about their own struggles and frustrations. One can be an advocate in one or more different situations, depending on the needs of the person who requires assistance. In order to determine these needs there are **Six Steps of Support** that one could take in determining how and when to apply for services to meet the needs of the person that they are representing.

Step One – Assessing the Required Services
Interviews with the Person with Mental Illness, family, friends and other caregivers will assist the Advocate in determining both immediate services and ongoing services

required. The Advocate and/or Supporter must be careful not to make their own assessment without consulting with others as sometimes that assessment could be based on wrong assumptions.

Step Two – Understanding Bureaucracy

Bureaucracy is well established in society's institutions and accessing the services, often hidden within the bureaucratic system, can be a challenge, to say the least. The Advocate's knowledge of how these systems work is an essential element to taking the first step in figuring out how and when the services can be obtained. This step involves learning the names, positions, duties and responsibilities of individuals who work in the system so that you don't waste time waiting until someone contacts you that actually cannot assist you.

Step Three – Documenting and Comparing Available Services

Based on the assessment in Step One, and Understanding Bureaucracy in Step Two including an inventory of "where to look and who to talk to", Step Three includes documenting the available services and comparing them to one another. For example, when searching for subsidized housing, the Supporter would list all the homeless shelters available on an emergency basis and/or for short stay periods, the rules and regulations regarding admittance to these shelters, and follow up programs once a person is discharged.

Step Four – Networking with Service Providers

Networking with Service Providers allows the Supporter to "put a name to a face", and connect with these providers in a positive manner. For example, this may include touring facilities, attending seminars that describe the programs, meeting persons who access the services, and obtaining the necessary administrative forms to apply for the services.

Step Five – Reconnecting with the Person with Mental Illness
At this point, the Supporter has considered the needs and wishes of the person requiring services, consulted with this person and others, analyzed where and when these services can be accessed, met with Service Providers, and compiled a concise report describing each service. The Supporter then takes the report to the Person with Mental Illness and carefully points out what is available, without pressuring this person to jump right in and agree to the Supporter's suggestions. Step Five can be the most difficult step of all. The person requiring service may not show any interest in the report, especially if they are suffering from Depression. If they are experiencing hypomania, it is likely they will feel they can handle everything on their own and don't need anyone's help. In a full blown manic state they may have disappeared or been admitted to psychiatric care in a Hospital.

It is crucial that the Supporter understands that patience is definitely a virtue. There will be a moment in time when a person is more willing to listen and agree to access services with the Supporter's assistance. In the meantime, the Supporter can continue to repeat the previous steps in order to remain updated on any changes.

Step Six – Follow-Up

Once a person requiring services starts to access and use these services the role of the Supporter does not end. Follow-up, evaluation, and regular contact with Service Providers is essential in order to iron out any glitches, and guide a person through roadblocks that may cause them to resist any further assistance. For example, if a person is receiving a government disability pension which requires an annual review, they may be too ill to take the form to their Physician for an evaluation. These annual reviews usually require medical documentation that confirms the person's Mental Illness as ongoing. The Supporter must be aware of the steps required to renew the disability benefits, the deadline for renewal, and gently guide the person through the process. Without this basic financial assistance, and without family support, too many people end up homeless. They live their life (and often a short life at that point) without any shelter, food or proper medications.

During Brent's manic episodes when he wandered through the streets of Vancouver my knowledge of the inner city shelters and connection with the staff who work there made it much easier for me to find him. Even though he didn't always come home with Bob and me he knew that we cared enough to keep up the search over and over again. There were also times when we did persuade him to go to the Hospital with us as he trusted our judgment even though the mania did not.

☙❧

In summary, the **Six Steps of Support**, although they may

be sequential at first as the Supporter attempts to assess and access services, can be revisited whenever necessary. During the follow-up phase the Supporter may go back to each and/or any of the other steps if further information is required. Often, the Supporter will consult with the person who requires the services to include them in the process.

The remainder of this chapter will apply the Six Steps to Support to the different services: Education, Community, Healthcare and Social Services, and Employment programs. As the Supporter goes through these steps it will become obvious that services are sometimes unavailable or difficult to access. There may be few, if any, services in a particular community due to geographical isolation, lack of proper healthcare facilities and programs, and the unwillingness of people to acknowledge that Mental Illness exists in their community. The Supporter will learn that part of the process involves lobbying the "movers and shakers", i.e. those who make political decisions, as well as educating the public on Mental Illness.

The importance of lobbying and ways to do just that will be discussed in the chapter, **"Hearing the Silent Voices"**.

EDUCATION

Mental Illness is being diagnosed more frequently at an earlier age such that children who show various symptoms may benefit from medical treatment and support services throughout their childhood. These symptoms, as they become more obvious, often make it difficult for a child to adapt to the classroom and the social environment in their school and community. The parent or parents will probably receive feedback from the Teacher that their child is showing one or more of the following symptoms: lack of concentration, withdrawing from interacting with other children or showing aggression towards them, not completing assignments, talking too much in class or not talking at all, obsessive-compulsive behaviors, restlessness, etc. At first, the Teacher may consult with the parents, ask for feedback and give suggestions as to how to assist the child in improving their performance in class as well as interact more appropriately with the other children. It is not uncommon for a Teacher to advise parents to take their child to a Physician for vision and hearing tests to determine if they need glasses and/or hearing aids. Medical tests could be given to rule out allergies and other physical conditions that might provoke inappropriate behavior.

Teachers and/or School Counselors can also refer a child to their school district's Special Services Program to be assessed for possible learning disabilities.

The parents may disclose that they are having difficulties at home such as illness in the family, divorce and custody disputes, and/or adjustment to a new baby. The School District Personnel, Teachers, and the caregivers can then devise a plan in which the child will be given the opportunity to express their feelings in a safe environment in order to disclose what is happening to them. Bullying in schools is a serious problem that is finally being recognized by the school system and the public. Often, if children are being threatened and bullied at school, they are too afraid to tell their Teachers or parents for fear of retribution by those who are bullying them.

Teachers may refer children to the School Counselors or call Child Protective Services to determine whether or not they are being subjected to neglect, physical, sexual and/or emotional abuse at home. The parents may become aware of interviews (after these interviews are completed in situations where the Teacher or other School Personnel suspect possible abuse), and can request a meeting with School Personnel to discuss the findings.

Step One: Assessing the Required Services

Once it has been determined that the child does not have physical problems such as poor vision or hearing, learning disabilities, is not a victim of bullying and/or neglect or abuse at home or in the community, one can then proceed to request an assessment of the child's mental health. This involves the participation of mental health resources, cooperation of the school, parents, and/or caregivers, and willingness on the part of the child to participate. This participation may consist of psychological tests, interviews with a Psychiatrist, and further medical tests as determined necessary by the child's Physician.

Assessing the required services, once all the interviews, tests, and consultations have been completed, becomes the Supporter's focus. The parents and/or the caregivers do not have to be the Supporter, especially if they decide that their emotional involvement makes it difficult for them to be objective. The parent(s) and/or caregiver(s) of the child can designate another family member, friend or community advocate to carry out the duties of the Supporter as objective analysis is necessary during this process. The Supporter could organize an assessment meeting involving all those who have participated in the assessment phase, and assist the group in pinpointing what resources are necessary to assist the child with mental health issues. It is important for the Supporter to stress to others that specific labeling of a Mental Illness would be premature at such an early age unless the completed tests and assessments have come up with an obvious diagnosis.

The Supporter's role in assisting an adult with mental health issues is no different than their role in assisting a child. The education system usually involves connection with Technical Institutes, Business Schools, Colleges, Universities, Trade Schools or Institutes, and other post-secondary institutions. Caregivers, School Personnel, Special Needs Instructors and Counselors, Physicians and Mental Health professionals all play a part in assisting the Supporter and the adult requesting further education. The person requesting educational opportunities may not have received proper diagnosis of their Mental Illness until Step One has been completed. In fact, it may come to light that the previous diagnosis has been incorrect, due to lack of research and information at the time of the original diagnosis or other problems overshadowing the Mental Illness such as Alcoholism and/or Drug Addiction.

At this point, the Supporter's role involves devising a preliminary educational plan with the person requesting more formal education based on the person's interests, skills, knowledge and challenges due to their mental health issues. This plan will be revised and updated according to the availability of programs in the person's geographical area, although more courses now are offered online by various Colleges and Universities.

The Supporter's main focus continues to be document-ing required services in a concise, clear format with the understanding that ongoing communication with the person requesting services remains a high priority. This com-munication is enhanced by face-to-face meetings where information is presented in a clear, positive manner to the person struggling with Mental Illness. Feedback from the person remains an integral part of the plan. No matter how discouraged or negative the feedback may be, it is feedback that must be considered, rather than minimized or dismissed. The trust between the Supporter and person requesting services will go a long way in assisting the per-son with their educational goals even when they appear to have little hope that they could achieve their goals because of their Mental Illness.

Step Two: Understanding Bureaucracy
Understanding bureaucracy does not have to be a difficult process. The Supporter does not need to waste time going through the phone book in order to find the appropriate ministry and/or department that may provide services. The most expedient way to find information is by contact-ing the administrative office of your local politician as they will have an assistant who handles public enquiries. These assistants are usually "up to speed" on the roles and re-sponsibilities of different government ministries and can refer the Supporter to the appropriate contact person in these ministries. As well, they will have a list of social ser-vice agencies and other community groups that offer pro-grams and services, and contact persons in these groups.

It can be very frustrating when one is put on hold on the

telephone or expected to go through several menus which often bring you back to the main menu. The contact person will likely have an email address, fax number, phone number and mailing address. Contact through email can be much faster as the Supporter has a written record of their attempts to obtain information. It is not always possible to arrange a face-to-face meeting, especially if the contact person is responsible for a large region, rather than one community. The Politician's Administrative Assistant will also assist the Supporter in getting action if the Supporter comes back with written proof of efforts to get information via email, fax, and/or mail. It is reasonable to wait 2 to 4 weeks for a response, try again, and then go back to the Administrative Assistant for further direction. If the Supporter has shown that they have made a reasonable effort to find information to no avail, the Assistant can brief the Politician on the problem, who, in turn, has the authority to check with the Ministry or other government personnel as to why there has been no response.

It is crucial that the Supporter work cooperatively with the Assistant in an assertive, pleasant manner to show them that they have made every effort to follow up on the information provided to them by the Assistant.

Access to a computer is a necessity these days as much information can be retrieved online, with names of contacts, phone numbers, email addresses, etc. Descriptions of programs and services are available, especially when the Supporter enters keywords that apply to the accessed services required. For example, if the assessment includes the need for special services for persons who want to attain high school equivalency keywords such as "high school equivalency — special needs" or "online high school up-grading — special services" may pinpoint exactly where to enquire in the government bureaucracy.

Face-to-face contact is still one of the most productive ways to nail down exactly what is available and through direct contact with the resource person the Supporter then has the opportunity to ask specific questions and request clarification of responses. As the Supporter compiles information they may have received online, through the mail, and/or by dropping by offices where services are provided, they can review this information and request a one-on-one interview with the contact person or resource person responsible for describing the educational programs and application process for these programs. The most effective way to narrow down the search is by preparing a brief, written report outlining educational services required and attaching a list of questions for the contact person. Send this report to the contact person in advance of the meeting so that they can prepare for the meeting as well. This also gives the contact person time to arrange for other personnel to sit in on the interview who may explain in more detail what is involved in registering for a specific educational program.

Contacting the different educational institutions and requesting an interview with the Financial Aid Department and/or Special Services for Students Program is advisable as the Supporter can explain the challenges facing the person with the Mental Illness to the contact person. The contact person may suggest certain programs and financial assistance available through their Special Services Program, and outline to the Supporter whether or not the educational program and financial assistance service is flexible should the person become ill and require a course extension.

Student loans, although often available, can be stressful to a Person with Mental Illness who often, is not employed, and do not feel confident that they could ever pay the loan back to the financial institution. Trade schools, Colleges, and Universities sometimes offer part-time studies with Special Needs grants to assist in the payment of tuition, student fees, and the purchase of textbooks and tutors' services. The Supporter should enquire under what terms and conditions these grants are available as that information is not easy for the public to find. The Supporter may also be able to negotiate terms and conditions of admission requirements by requesting flexibility in attendance, process for handling absenteeism and make-up sessions should the person experience a relapse of their illness. The more these issues are discussed up front and dealt with, the greater the chance of success of the Person with Mental Illness completing their program.

Step 3: Documenting and Comparing Available Services
The Supporter will now have an inventory of different educational programs, where they are offered, financial assistance available, and admission requirements. It is useful to draw a chart with columns that assist the Supporter in comparing the programs and explaining them to the person requesting them. It becomes quite evident which programs offer the most flexibility, financial grants, and courses relevant to the interests and goals outlined in Step One. Geographical proximity is a key factor as long com-

mutes to and from school often adds more stress to the daily routine. A Person with Mental Illness may find it difficult to be in crowds for long periods on public transit or sit in rush hour traffic two to three hours a day. Part-time studies, one or two courses at a time, with flexibility built in to extend a course of studies when acute phases of the illness occur, will also increase the chances of a person's successful completion of studies.

A Person with Mental Illness can also take non-credit courses through continuing studies in educational institutes and/or night school and weekend programs offered by Municipal Governments, High Schools, and Community Organizations. These courses will give them the opportunity to pursue hobbies and volunteer activities that assist them in developing and enhancing their knowledge, skills, and abilities. Sometimes the completion of non-credit courses gives a person confidence to pursue credit programs that may lead to employment. The Supporter will not find it difficult to obtain various leisure guides and continuing studies brochures from the local Municipal Hall, Community Centre, and Parks and Recreation Departments. They can outline what is available to the Person with Mental Illness based on the assessment in Step One. It is not uncommon for the non-credit programs to also offer grants or subsidies based on financial need. Regional Government Programs may offer public transit passes and/or specialized transportation services at a reduced rate also based on financial need.

The Supporter's organization of material in a systematic, concise manner goes a long way in assisting a Person with Mental Illness to determine what program(s) they would be willing to consider. The Supporter may find it useful to purchase a three ring binder with titles such as Financial Assistance, Recreation Interests and Hobbies, Self-Improvement Courses, Post-Secondary Education Programs, Special Services, and Resource Persons. Although the person requesting service should have their own copy, it is the role of the Supporter to ensure that the manual is updated on a regular basis. Each time there is a change and/or addition to the manual the Supporter can take the opportunity to meet with the person requesting service and review their goals and objectives at that time.

Step Four: Networking with Service Providers

Networking with Service Providers is an ongoing process. Once the manual has been compiled for the first time, the Supporter can continue to make contact with Service Providers for updates. In addition, the Supporter will likely have a more realistic view if they tour facilities, attend seminars that address specific programs and clarify procedures required for admission. The Supporter may have listed several programs in the manual based on the interests of the person requesting further education. They will then be better prepared to describe the education programs by touring the facilities and interviewing Coordinators and Resource Persons attached to the programs.

Genuine concern shown by the Supporter often encourages resource persons to "go the extra mile" for students who require special services and consideration in order to pursue their studies. Although there are rules and procedures to follow in any institution, there is also flexibility when resource persons are committed to open, accessible education for everyone, including those with health issues. This commitment can be reinforced by face-to-face contact between the Supporter, resource person and the person requesting admission to a post-secondary institution.

Step Five: Reconnecting with the Person with Mental Illness
The Supporter may feel enthusiastic in that they have compiled a detailed manual of education programs available according to the needs and interest assessment completed in Step One. However, the Person with Mental Illness doesn't always share that enthusiasm if they have enrolled in a program in the past but couldn't complete it due to their illness. They may not be receptive to enrolling again if they are presented with a plan while they are experiencing depression, mania, and/or hallucinations and delusions. The Supporter must be patient and present the educational opportunities during a relatively stable period. Other volunteer community programs can be presented as a "stepping stone" to further post-secondary education. A review of needs and interests established in Step One is necessary in case other medical issues or life circumstances have occurred since the initial assessment.

Reconnecting can also include a tour of the educational institute that has been selected as the first choice, and a meeting with the Program Coordinator who may have already met the Supporter, where the specifics of the program are outlined to the person requesting the service. The Supporter plays a useful role here in the background where they encourage the Person with Mental Illness to ask questions directly of the Program Coordinator. If the Person with Mental Illness has chosen to get involved in non-credit courses and/or volunteer work, tours and meetings can also be arranged for the purpose of clarifying admission procedures and discussing flexible terms and conditions.

The Supporter will likely present their information to a person requesting educational programs in an initial meeting and revisit this information with them once they have had a chance to consider their options. It may take several sessions before the Person with Mental Illness is ready to apply to a particular program but this does not mean that they aren't interested. They have often experienced too many setbacks in their lives that add to their poor self-esteem and resulting despair. The Supporter must continue to emphasize that Mental Illness is not their fault. Each effort to improve their lives may be two steps forward and one step back, but eventually they will become more confident each time they succeed in their efforts.

Step Six: Follow-up

This is the final step in Six Steps of Support. This can be accomplished by regular check-ins with resource persons who manage each of the educational programs selected by the Person with Mental Illness. Keep updated on post-secondary educational special services, financial grants, scholarships, and be wary of student loan programs. The manual will need regular inserts as new information becomes available and contact data of resource persons changes depending on these persons moving to other employment. This follow-up often includes visits to the Hospital if and when the Person with Mental Illness suffers a relapse. Not only will the Supporter show unconditional support by visiting them but must also contact the Education Contact Person and request an extension of the program studies. If a Physician's note is required the Supporter can arrange for that through the Hospital Social Worker or Community Liaison Personnel. The message that "this relapse is not your fault; your educational studies have not been cancelled, just postponed until you have recovered" goes a long way in giving a person in the Psychiatric Ward even a little ray of hope. Hope, through Compassion and Despair is never more important than when a person lies in a Psychiatric Hospital bed blaming themselves for their relapse.

As the Supporter reviews this **Six Steps of Support** they may feel overwhelmed with the requirement involved in completing each step. However, a systematic approach will produce positive results and continuous follow-up will make it easier to follow these steps as new challenges face the Supporter and the person they are assisting. Education is life-long learning and each accomplishment, whether it is volunteer work, self-improvement, and/or completion of non-credit and for credit courses, connects each of us with our environment and community. It decreases the sense of isolation and loneliness so often felt by persons suffering from Mental Illness.

COMMUNITY: HEALTHCARE AND SOCIAL SERVICES

Step One: Assessing the Required Services
The process involved in accessing Healthcare and Social Services is similar to that of accessing Educational Services.

However, this time, others will be involved as well as the Person with Mental Illness. The Supporter may determine that this person needs medical attention, assistance in acquiring and taking medications, hospitalization followed by re-entry in to the community such as short-term group home placement, out-Patient programs, and gradual return to their accommodations and daily life. The person's accommodations may need housekeeping services, fresh groceries, and payment of bills such as rent, utilities, phone, and cable. The Supporter may provide these services themselves if they have access to the person's accommodations or they may coordinate these services with the person's family members and friends. A small gesture of support can make a difference when a person returns to their home after Hospitalization to find a clean apartment with food in the fridge and cupboards, rather than rotting garbage, spoiled food, and a dark apartment.

On different occasions while Brent was in Hospital my family has assisted me in cleaning his apartment and replenishing his supplies. He trusts Bob and I with a key and his bankcard at those times so that he doesn't spend the little money that he has by withdrawing cash from the ATM machine in the Hospital. We are also able to enter his apartment, remove the garbage and clutter in his suite and pay his bills from his bank account. During manic episodes, as mentioned earlier, Brent will pick up so much stuff that one can hardly move in his apartment. I have sorted through this stuff carefully and consulted with him as to what I could reorganize, recycle or throw away while he was in the Hospital. This consultation works best when his mania is subsiding and he willingly accepts our

119

intervention. Other family members have assisted as well. For example, his Aunt Lesley has helped me clean up his apartment, and his sister has rearranged his furniture to create more space, put up shelves, and painted various items for him.

During past manic episodes Brent signed up for magazine subscriptions whenever he came across salespersons offering a free trial. As a Supporter I obtained Brent's permission to open his mail when he was in Hospital, and followed up by writing to several companies regarding his condition. I explained to these companies (in writing) that Brent lives on a disability pension and cannot afford these subscriptions; they complied in every instance, stopped requesting payments, and honored my request to cancel the subscriptions.

A Person with Mental Illness may not have friends and/or family members to assist them in determining what type of healthcare and social services are necessary. The Supporter, in this case, can consult with the Psychiatrist, Hospital Social Worker, Hospital Nurses, Mental Health Nurses, Community Social Workers, and Community Physician. This consultation can only be done with the written permission of the Person with Mental Illness which is not always easy to acquire. As explained earlier in this chapter, gaining the person's trust on an ongoing basis is crucial to obtaining this permission, and goes a long way to assessing their needs and coordinating the required services to meet these needs. During Brent's most recent manic episode, I arranged with the Mental Health Social Worker and the Hospital Psychiatrist for Brent to be discharged from Hospital and reside in a short-term Boarding

Home Program. Brent's mania had subsided enough for him to be admitted to the Boarding Home and he agreed to comply with their rules and regulations. He was also included in a preliminary meeting where the rules were explained by the Social Worker who, fortunately, had good rapport with Brent. This worker was a gentle man who treated Brent as an adult, with dignity and respect. He did not talk down to Brent or act in a condescending manner towards him. He listened carefully to Brent's concerns and answered his questions directly, rather than ignoring him, and did not make comments and suggestions to Bob and me as if Brent was not present at the meeting.

"Transition" meetings just before discharge from Hospital should include discussions on the following:

- *Hospital out-Patient programs,*

- *Medications required with a process in place to phone in medications to a pharmacy familiar with a person's previous medications,*

- *Community programs such as Mental Health Drop-in Centers,*

- *Follow-up meetings with Mental Health Worker, and acknowledgement that the Supporter will act as liaison between Hospital and Person with Mental Illness should a reoccurrence of the illness result in another Hospital stay. These meetings should include the Person with Mental Illness, and involve discussions of all the services that are available to this person once they are discharged.*

Although Hospital Psychiatric Programs usually have a discharge meeting, without the Supporter coordinating the efforts of all those involved, the patient may attend the meeting without actually participating. Too often they remain passive, anxious to be discharged, and not responsive to any treatment plan proposed by the Hospital staff. A treatment plan without the input of the patient usually "falls on deaf ears". The Supporter can ensure that the patient's needs are represented and that the treatment plan is based on the patient's needs and personal situation. One size does not fit all!

Step Two: Understanding Bureaucracy

This step may be difficult for the Supporter in the health care system. The location of social services are easier to find in that they are offered by non-profit societies, churches, local governments, service clubs, and Hospital out-Patient programs. However, specific healthcare services are not widely advertised by Regional, Provincial and Federal Governments even if general services are advertised in pamphlets and brochures. One can find a list of specific services by visiting non-profit societies in their community and arranging for an appointment with the staff. These non-profit societies may receive some or most of their funding from government health departments or ministries. Their staff will explain to the Supporter the services provided by their organization as well as those services provided directly by government. They will also help the Supporter "fast track" their way to finding the information they require from the healthcare system. The same approach that was explained in accessing the educational system can be applied to accessing the healthcare system.

Mental health agencies are also connected to the healthcare bureaucracy and the staff in those agencies can help the Supporter navigate their way to finding healthcare services. The Supporter must come to these meetings prepared with questions and a description of services assessed in Step One. If staff does not have the time to meet with a Supporter, talk to their supervisor, and request a meeting with someone who can provide answers. Telephone interviews or email conversations can be useful in obtaining information but there are times when face-to-face meetings are necessary to grasp a complete understanding of how to navigate through a bureaucracy. These meetings will help the Supporter achieve relevant answers to their questions as well as a list of contact persons and "the inside track" on how to reach them for further information. The inside track is the unwritten guidelines to accessing the bureaucracy; i.e. the "human element" that comes in to play when applying for and receiving government healthcare services.

Step Three: Documenting and Comparing Available Healthcare and Social Services

This step is a reality check for the Supporter. At this stage the cost of acquiring any of these services can become problematic for the Person with Mental Illness. For example, the person's benefit plan through their income assistance or disability pension often covers only part of the costs for medications, dental work, and other extended services such as vision care, hearing aids, physiotherapy, massage therapy, etc. The Supporter can make a diligent effort to "dig deeper" by requesting more information on subsidies available to assist with these costs. It never fails to amaze me how quiet some government personnel can be on letting the public know that subsidies are available. In cases where certain prescription medications are not covered, some government medical programs allow those medications to be covered if the Physician writes up a special order. The Supporter would let the Physician know that their patient requires this special order as they cannot afford to purchase the prescription drugs necessary to monitor and treat their Mental Illness.

Income assistance rates and disability pensions do not increase enough to meet the needs of those requiring financial assistance. Often, these rates are frozen for years and as healthcare costs increase, the income of the Person with Mental Illness does not meet their basic cost of living, never mind healthcare costs. Various healthcare agencies offer reduced rates for those who cannot afford the going rate. They are able to do so because some Physicians, Dentists, and other medical professionals donate time to providing these services. The Supporter now compares different programs they have discovered in Step Two, and investigates further as to where the special subsidies are offered and by whom. With the permission of the person requiring services the Supporter can help them fill out the paperwork, arrange for the appointments, and accompany them or coordinate friends or family to accompany them to their appointments.

Comparison of social service programs is important, especially the requirements of these programs for someone to access what is available to them. Most food banks have policies as to how often a person can receive food, and whether or not they have to meet a financial means test. It can be humiliating for anyone to stand in line for groceries, meals, and other necessities. The person in need of these programs may find it too stressful to do just that. The Supporter can explain the policies to them, assist them in applying at first for the services, and in some cases, with certain food banks, pick up the groceries for the person. The Supporter will get a strong sense of the attitude of Service Providers by speaking to the staff and touring the facilities. The "way" in which persons requiring these services are treated is just as important as receiving the basics, such as food, clothing, and shelter.

Programs that allow for a person requiring services to also volunteer in these or other community programs assist them in giving back to their community. The Supporter's comparison of all programs must include a column on attitude of resource persons, in addition to type of service, geographical location and accessibility, financial cost, frequency, and relevancy to assessment of services required, outlined in Step One.

At this stage, the Supporter will have compiled a list of the those healthcare and social services required by the Person with Mental Illness, as well as outlined a comparison of these services. The outline should contain a timeline with the most urgent services highlighted as priorities.

Step Four: Networking with Service Providers
Now the Supporter is ready to nail down exactly what is required to obtain the services as soon as possible. The

Supporter may have toured the facilities and reviewed the social service programs face to face with Service Providers.

In terms of healthcare programs the process is usually more formal, and networking with those who can fast track the process is essential to acquiring healthcare services in a timely manner. Completion of necessary paperwork is essential to avoid unnecessary delays in receiving services. The wheels of bureaucracy move slowly, and as the expression goes "the squeaky wheel gets the grease". Supporters can be "squeaky" in an assertive way but will only alienate Service Providers if they show their frustration by being aggressive towards them. Networking means showing respect for those who have the information and appreciating their support throughout the process.

Step Five: Reconnecting with the Person with Mental Illness
Reconnecting with a Person with Mental Illness may include intervention by the Supporter in a crisis situation where hospitalization and emergency medical attention is necessary. The person suffering from a relapse may agree to voluntarily admit themselves to the Psychiatric Ward in order to stabilize their condition. However, the Supporter may have to persuade the Emergency Physician to agree to admit a person who may appear rational at the time of the interview in the Emergency Ward. Too often, if psychiatric beds are not available, a person suffering from Depression who does not admit that they are feeling suicidal may get sent home. The Supporter can insist on admittance as soon as the next bed is available while in the meantime try to arrange for 24 hour supervision at home with family and

friends. If the person requesting voluntary admittance has no support systems the Supporter must explain this to the Physician on duty, and emphasize that this person needs to be admitted, even if it means remaining in emergency until a bed becomes available.

An acute, psychotic breakdown usually requires medical certification by one or more Physicians, depending on the Mental Health Act in the person's province or state. The Supporter needs to be familiar with this legislation and any other related legislation that outline the rights of persons suffering from Mental Illness. I have taken a copy of this legislation with me to show Hospital personnel that I understand patients' rights, and the procedure required regarding voluntary and involuntary admission. Brent has given me permission in several situations to act on his behalf, and at those times, I have the right to request written documentation from the Hospital pertaining to the certification process. The more the Supporter knows about the correct procedures and shares this knowledge with medical professionals, the greater the chances that service will not only be quicker but be within the parameters of what the Hospital staff is permitted to carry out as a treatment plan for the patient.

If intervention is not required at Step 5, the Supporter can share the list of available healthcare and social services to a person requiring additional help. Keep in mind that this person may be reluctant to accept what they perceive as "handouts", and may feel ashamed, embarrassed or humiliated that they even need assistance. No matter how hard the Supporter tries to reassure a person that their Mental Illness is the reason they are having difficulty working, participating in community activities, and taking care of their own needs on a daily basis, Persons with Mental Illness often blame themselves. The stigma of Mental Illness is "alive and well in our world", and will only be reduced and hopefully eliminated as society becomes better educated and more willing to embrace the responsibility of eradicating such a devastating illness.

In the meantime, the Supporter must continue to reintroduce their inventory of services again in the hopes that the person they are trying to help will accept some form of assistance.

Step Six: Follow-up

Follow-up is an ongoing process as the Supporter revisits resource persons and facilities, and removes roadblocks that arise during intervention or implementation of services. Healthcare services may initially be a "one time only" service with short-term deadlines to apply for temporary assistance. The Supporter can find out the process involved in extending these services, and help a person reapply for them. Letters signed by Physicians confirming the medical diagnosis of a person's illness are necessary to show that the illness is chronic, even if a person is stable for long periods of time. Until there is a cure for all forms of Mental Illness a person requiring service should not be seen as "cured" just because they have not been hospitalized for some time. The Supporter has to remind Service Providers that the illness is there everyday, even if it is not always obvious to society at large.

Inclusion of the Person with Mental Illness during Step Six is an integral part of the Supporter's role in that the

Supporter must never lose sight that they are assisting and encouraging this person to improve their life, even when they feel their life has been wasted on their illness. Follow-up involves assistance with the completion of the following administrative tasks:

- *Filling out application forms,*

- *Acquiring medical documentation,*

- *Filling prescriptions,*

- *Arranging life skills courses,*

- *Applying for volunteer work,*

- *Registering for "fast-track" Hospitalization,*

- *Registering for Out-Patient programs.*

The Supporter may intervene when it is critical, but then needs to retreat once a person accepting services begins to seek help on their own. At that point, the Supporter remains in the background, always available for consultation and support should this person ask for further assistance and/or intervention.

EMPLOYMENT SERVICES

Employment Services for Persons with Mental Illness are difficult to find. Society has not yet accepted the terms and conditions necessary to accommodate the challenges of Mental Illness and to embrace the value in providing meaningful work to those who struggle daily with their illness. Yes, there are pre-employment programs in some communities that offer job readiness such as workplace etiquette, how to write a resume, job search techniques, and preparing for an interview. These programs are short-term, of course, and even though there may be built-in flexibility while attending them, they are not set up to assist a person in handling the challenges they will face as the symptoms of their illness are manifested in the workplace.

Step One: Assessing Employment Services

This assessment will not take long as there are not many services out there. The list for educational and volunteer programs, healthcare services, and community social services discussed previously in this chapter will be much longer than employment services. Yet, so many Persons with Mental Illness continue to express a desire to work and to contribute to society by earning an income that can help them pay their own way.

During the time that the Supporter has compiled a manual of other services it will become apparent that some of the educational institutes, government departments, and non-profit societies are linked to pre-vocational and vocational services. Resource persons will give the Supporter contact information and probably an opinion of how effective these programs are for persons seeking flexibility and accommodation in the workplace. One does not look at glossy brochures outlining goals and objectives of employment programs designed to find employment for persons with disabilities, only to discover that few placements are long-term; nor do they always include work that is meaningful to those who try these opportunities.

Interviews with Persons with Mental Illness regarding their employment interests, skills, and abilities are necessary in order to seek employment programs and/or jobs that match as closely as possible the assessment attained from these interviews. Safety issues are paramount here as daily medications may rule out certain vocations. Recommendations from the person's Psychiatrist can assist in the assessment if they point out what job placements might lead to workplace injuries due to impairments brought on by side effects of the medications. The Supporter can also arrange for the person requesting employment to attend a pre-vocational assessment program, if one is available in their area, in order to determine their knowledge, skills, and abilities. An inventory of these skills may be drawn up at this program that show a Person with Mental Illness that they can contribute, even if they don't have a resume with credentials such as post-education degrees and previous employment.

Step Two: Understanding Bureaucracy

Bureaucratic procedures that are necessary to follow in order to assist a person seeking employment can be slow, tedious, and frustrating for the Supporter as they attempt to find out timelines, requirements for admissions, financial costs, etc. One must persevere through the process, checking with contact persons along the way. Check with your Federal Government Employment Office and request a face to face interview with the manager as that person should know exactly what programs are available to Persons with Special Needs. If the manager states that you don't need to meet with them, i.e., they will send you information, ask for name of their manager and stress the importance of face-to-face meetings. Someone in the government bureaucracy has a responsibility to meet with Persons with Mental Illness and/or their advocates and explain the goals and objectives of each program. If they are not qualified to do this they should refer you to others who specialize in programs designed to accommodate special needs, and outline financial grants, bursaries, and loans available to those in financial need.

One important question to ask once a person completes a pre-vocational program, on the job training, and/or other apprenticeship opportunities, is "what is the obligation of the employer to accommodate their special needs"? The manager or resource person will be able to answer this question if their federal program is providing financial assistance to employers. They can also can refer you to someone else who liaisons between employers and employees with special needs.

Step Three: Documenting and Comparing Employment Services
Once your assessment is complete, and you have a good understanding of government employment programs that might be useful, it is time to proceed to Step Three and Step Four. You will have met with Service Providers already when you assessed educational, healthcare, and social services in your community. These same resource persons often connect you to specialists who arrange for employment services. Again, the Supporter must ask the hard questions: "will this employment opportunity be cancelled if an employee has a relapse of their illness; is there a liaison available to assist the employee and employer

if and when issues arise in the workplace; are other employees aware of workplace challenges facing those suffering from Mental Illness"? When the Supporter compares available services they should consider the following factors: employer's flexibility to accommodate special needs, liaison persons to deal with crisis and other issues that arise in the workplace, education programs available to all employees on myths and facts of Mental Illness, sick leave and other benefits, employer evaluations, part-time opportunities, wages, and opportunities for advancement according to the person's challenges rather than "one size fits all".

Most important of all, the current day workplace culture of **WORK HARDER, WORK FASTER, WORK SMARTER,** adopted by so many companies and organizations driven to achieve, is unhealthy for all employees. This philosophy creates undue stress in the workplace. Not only does it increase sick leave and poor morale but decreases productivity.

Step Four: Networking with Employment Resource Persons

Persons with Mental Illness will be set up to fail if they enter a workplace poisoned with this "hard driving, achieve at all costs" mantra. The Supporter will soon discover what employment services and programs need to be avoided. Networking with Service Providers, touring worksites, interviewing prospective employers, and "asking around", will assist the Supporter to include in the manual those vocational services that value their employees, operate within a spirit of inclusion, and accommodate special needs. These employers, shareholders of companies, and other investors must be willing to make less of a profit in order to provide opportunities for those who want to contribute and pay their own way in life as much as possible. To put it simply, "it is the right thing to do".

Step Five: Reconnecting to a Person with Mental Illness

Reconnecting to a Person with Mental Illness in order to discuss possible pre-employment programs, employment services, and/or work opportunities requires the Supporter to present a clear, well-organized summary of vocational areas to pursue. This can be difficult in that it is not unusual for a person who is trying to cope on a day-to-day basis to lose faith that they will ever be able to find and sustain gainful employment. The Supporter can assist this person by presenting a realistic view of how to enter the workforce. A gradual entry in to the workplace will allow a person time to learn to manage the increased stress they may feel by having to meet the expectations of their employer and co-workers. Proper orientation and training on the worksite at a reasonable pace (where the person has time to ask questions and request clarification as well as check in with their liaison contact) will help them gain confidence.

Step Six: Follow-Up

Follow-up comes in to play as the Supporter's contact with the employer representative and/or liaison person will help to resolve conflicts and clear up misunderstandings that might arise in the workplace.

I encourage Supporters to pursue part-time employment opportunities for persons requesting entry or reentry in to the workforce. This does not mean that full-time employment is not an option; rather, in situations where stress is greatly increased by the pressures of full-time duties, these situations may trigger a relapse of the illness. Also, a person's disability pension or financial assistance services may allow the person to earn additional income up to a certain point. After that, the financial assistance could be reduced and eventually eliminated. Although this may seem okay if the person earns enough or more money than the financial assistance, it can become a crisis if and when the person is unable to work due to illness. It can be very difficult to reinstate financial assistance quickly as there is always, in my opinion, too much red tape that takes too long. The person, in the meantime, finds themselves financially destitute which only adds to the gravity of their relapse.

It is important for the Supporter to emphasize that work is valuable, whether it be part-time or full-time. It is the quality of the work that counts, not the quantity, and even though our North American culture places too much emphasis on "achieving and earning money", that does not mean that we should aspire to work in such a frenzy, where we are motivated by accumulating more and more material goods, at the expense of our health and our environment. A Person with Mental Illness may feel a greater sense of failure if they are trying to fit into the "rat race", a race that can make healthy people ill, and a race that could destroy our planet by depleting all of our resources. A proper health and safety procedure at work includes the creation of a harmonious and tolerant workplace environment. Education programs that explains the myths and facts of Mental Illness and other disabilities to employees and employers will go a long way to promoting tolerance and acceptance of those persons with disabilities who want to work The most effective programs emphasize the abilities of people, not the disabilities.

RELIABLE BUSINESS OF OUTSOURCING (Fraser Valley) and ABILITIES PLUS OUTSOURCING (Vancouver) are employment services in British Columbia, Canada that connect qualified contractors/consultants (with long term health issues) with local businesses that outsource administrative, technical and professional work on a contractual basis. This service points out that "this unique matching and placement service speaks directly to the needs of those who, after many years in the workforce, face a chronic health issue that compromises their ability to continue in full time traditional employment". Reliable Business Outsourcing is delivered in the Fraser Valley by Community Futures South Fraser and Abilities Plus Outsourcing by the ConnecTra Society, under the umbrella of the Sam Sullivan Disability Foundation in Vancouver. Their employment strategy views persons with challenges as having abilities that can be utilized by prospective employers on a contract basis, and that matches can be made between the contractor and contractee that are mutually beneficial. They outline their strategy and mandate as follows:

> *"We understand that professionals with health issues desire to contribute to society in a meaningful and productive way, while managing their physical, emotional and financial wellbeing. We also understand that businesses*

need access to a skilled flexible workforce on a short or long-term contract basis so we developed a strategy to partner these two groups for their mutual benefits.

Our mandate:

- *Develop a social enterprise that connects contractors/consultants to businesses' outsourcing needs;*

- *Build on existing relationships with multiple community sectors;*

- *Create a seamless service framework;*

- *Advance the self-employment of contractors/consultants with disabilities;*

- *Make a difference in people's lives.*

We value:

- *Skills of contractors with lifestyle needs;*

- *Community participation;*

- *Input from advisory committees and a network of business partners;*

- *Ethical business practices;*

- *The integrity of local business;*

- *Diversity of the entrepreneurial culture.*[3]

Funding partners which support this innovative, progressive employment service include Vancouver Foundation –

Disability Employment Support Fund, Vancity Credit Union, and sponsors include Western Economic Diversification Canada – Entrepreneurs with Disabilities Fund and Community Futures Development Association of BC.

This program/service assists individuals with health issues (health issue defined as "any continuous or recurrent condition — visible or not, that presents a barrier to competitive employment. It can be physical, sensory, learning, or mental health impairment), by preparing them for prospective employment as outlined above. Their assistance consists of "identifying their competencies, saleable expertise and specific contract area; effectively marketing and promoting their skills and services; using a streamlined match and placement process; negotiating a fair market rate for their services, and offering advice and follow-up support." In addition, the service supports contractors/consultants with skills and aptitude assessments, skills development workshops, business coaching and mentoring, group sessions, networking, liaison and support.

The program was initiated by Community Futures South Fraser which is a not-for-profit community-operated organization that provides leadership and support for business by nurturing local economic and entrepreneurial development, and acts as a catalyst to improve the social, cultural and economic well-being of the Abbotsford-Chilliwack, British Columbia area. For further information, contact Community Futures South Fraser at the following address:

#100, 32383 South Fraser Way,
Abbotsford, BC

V2T1W7

Phone # 604-864-5770

Email @ www.cfdscosf@southfraser.com

www.southfraser.com

Reliable Business Outsourcing can be contacted at the following:

Phone # 604-864-5770

Toll free #1-877-827-8249

www.reliable@southfraser.com

www.reliableoutsourcing.ca

Abilities Plus Outsourcing, based in Vancouver, B.C. can be contacted at the following:

Phone # 604-688-6464, extension 128

www.kduncan@connectra.org

The accommodation of disabilities in the workplace must be made, where necessary. **Step Six, Follow-Up,** must be an integral, ongoing part of the workplace experience for Persons with Mental Illness. Regular meetings to discuss achievements, areas that need improvement, workplace training and education programs, and ways to improve interpersonal communication will increase the probability of a successful work experience for all the employees and employer representatives. Emergency systems must be in place in case of a medical crisis with debriefing and counseling available to employees during and after the initial crisis has passed.

The Supporter also plays an important role in assisting a

person's return to work. A gradual return to work involves a process whereby the Supporter and/or liaison worker, employee and employer representative discuss necessary requirements to make the return to work successful. The groups will likely review written recommendations from medical professionals in order to determine what type of accommodations is required, and for what period of time. The employee must be cleared to return to work by their Physician before an employer is willing to allow them back to the workplace. The most common return to work program includes implementing accommodations, worksite orientation, and gradual increase of hours over several weeks. Check-ins with employees as to how they are doing could happen on a weekly or bi-weekly basis and adjustments made to actual tasks and hours of work, if necessary.

The Supporter must also ensure that necessary paperwork is completed so that a person in acute crisis can access sick leave and other medical benefits without facing undue financial hardship. A gradual return to work program is just as important as the initial placement at work, as relapses are a way of life for Persons with Mental Illness. Until there is a cure for all types of Mental Illness, employers must include these relapses as part of their workplace adjustment plan, rather than avoid hiring Persons with Mental Illness because they cannot guarantee that they will never miss a day of work.

Assisting a person requesting employment, helping them build enough confidence to actually apply for and accept a position, and providing follow-up services gives the Supporter the opportunity to build a bridge between a Person with Mental Illness and their community, and walk alongside this person as they cross that bridge. No matter how difficult the journey, the Supporter must never underestimate how much they, themselves, have contributed along the way.

The Importance of Community Programs and Employment Services

How often have many of us heard that people who are homeless want to live that way, and that they don't want any help. I feel annoyed and frustrated when I hear these comments although some people that make these comments may feel embarrassed or guilty because they just don't know how to help. They may have encountered someone on the street panhandling for money or sleeping on a sidewalk while they were walking to a concert or the theatre in the downtown core of a large city. Someone might have jumped in front of their car at a stoplight and started to wash their windshield, hoping for money in exchange for their un-solicited services. I do not see persons asking for food or money as lazy or unmotivated to support themselves. They are working hard at trying to survive, moment by moment. Sitting on a cement sidewalk, cap in hand, soaking wet or freezing cold is dangerous, hard work. Jumping in front of a car waiting at a traffic light to wash a windshield for small change is also dangerous for everyone involved. No one can convince me that anyone in this situation wants to be there, rather than have food, clothing, decent housing, and meaningful work in their lives. Too often Persons with Mental Illness, without support systems, have nowhere to go. The inner city may provide some emergency shel-ters, food banks, and of course, easy access to alcohol and drugs. It is not uncommon for Persons with Mental Illness to turn to alcohol and drugs in an attempt to cover up their pain and despair. The relationship between Mental Illness and Addictions is becoming more obvious, and progressive treatment programs are acknowledging this relationship as they work with clients who are seeking help.

The Supporter will have discovered during their assessment of services that basic services such as decent housing, pre-employment programs, and support groups are lacking in many communities. They will also be amazed at how many individuals, churches, non-profit societies, and service clubs are providing services wherever and whenever possible. There are pockets of services here and there run by countless volunteers who are trying to make a difference. However, the coordination of such services is not always possible as resources depend on long-term funding. Most funding is offered on a short-term basis and organizations have to compete for these funds. It is ironic that casino and gambling monies are made available to these groups and that some of these monies come from people who lose their money over and over again at the casinos. People with gambling addictions may seek addictions counseling from counselors whose wages are partially paid by monies lost by these same persons.

In my community social service agencies, churches, and politicians sit on a committee to acquire land and erect housing for persons who are homeless. It wasn't too long ago that only a few people were speaking to this issue, often to deaf ears. However, after several summers with 200 or more people sleeping in the parks, abandoned houses, and parking lots the complaints by local businesses and residents increased. Community parks attracted people who were dealing in drugs and local residents viewed the exchange of drugs on a daily basis. Public outcry was expressed through letters to the editor, delegations to local government council meetings, community groups, and provincial government representatives. The public reaction was mixed as some viewed the "homeless" as young kids who didn't want to obey rules at home or work for a living. I recall from my experiences as a Social Worker and Community Service Worker that young persons sometimes fled from their homes because they were being sexually, physically, and/or emotionally abused. They were not always believed by adults and without this acknowledgement by the authorities, the young people would take to the streets to escape the abuse at home. Others were showing signs of Mental Illness (often are manifested during puberty) and were kicked out of their homes because of their unpredictable, inappropriate behaviour.

There are single parents with children who are denied income assistance. There are families where the main provider has lost their job, used up their employment insurance benefits, and been evicted from their housing because they could no longer pay their rent. Ongoing support services are absolutely necessary to get these people back on track, and our society has a responsibility to build into our social safety net an ongoing commitment to provide and sustain these services. The hit and miss approach which includes short-term funding, often for programs that are short-staffed and short-lived, does not build a sustainable, healthy public service network. I believe we are our "brother's and sister's keeper", as at any moment in time those of us who are blessed with emotional stability could be faced with Mental Illness in our family and amongst our friends.

Employment opportunities, as mentioned earlier, must operate on the philosophy that meaningful work based on one's abilities, not disabilities, is important for Persons with Mental Illness to feel valued in the workplace. Disabilities must be accommodated with emphasis on training, liaison programs, and health and safety measures to deal with medical issues. These opportunities can include part-time employment that allow a Person with Mental Illness time to pace themselves, to handle stress more effectively, and to supplement their financial assistance with enough earnings and benefits to meet their living expenses.

Ongoing community support services, in addition to volunteer and/or employment, will reduce a person's sense of isolation and allow them to access public services with dignity and respect. Long-term funding through joint government, community and business initiatives will provide the stability needed to enhance the quality of these services provided by both staff and volunteers.

In my community a local society, **Stepping Stones Community Services**, not only provides a drop-in centre for Persons with Mental Illness, but involves the members in day-to-day running of the centre. It includes members in group discussions and planning sessions regarding services required. The members' input has raised the profile of Persons with Mental Illness in our community in a positive way as the public's awareness of the abilities of these persons has increased dramatically over the last ten years. This public awareness helps to build a new base of community support that goes a long way to ensuring continued and additional community support services as well as meaningful employment.

9

HEARING THE SILENT VOICES

The silent voices of Persons with Mental Illness may be a deafening roar inside their minds but only whispers to others close by. The Supporter as advocate listens quietly to each whisper and tries to bridge the gap between those who aren't able to speak and those who want to listen. The Supporter also encourages persons with silent voices to speak out for themselves through the written word, conversation in self-help support groups, participation in community education forums, and other media such as music, theatre, dance, volunteer activities, etc. **VISIONS,** a journal distributed by British Columbia's (Canada) Partners for Mental Health and Addictions Information, provides "a forum for the voices of people living with a mental disorder or substance use problem, their family and friends, and Service Providers in BC. VISIONS is written by and for people who have used mental health or addictions services (also known as consumers), family and friends, mental health and addictions Service Providers, providers from various other sectors, and leaders and decision-makers in the field. It creates a place where many perspectives on mental health and addictions issues can be heard."[4]

The **VISIONS** journal includes descriptions of addictions, treatment programs, research development and lists of resources and support services in the province. BC Partners receives financial support from the Provincial Health Services Authority and is an excellent example of how government and community organizations can cooperate in educating the public on mental health and addictions programs and services. **VISIONS** provide a venue for focus on special topics in each publication. For example, spring, 2006 issue features Alcohol and alternatives approaches to treatment. Winter, 2006, issue features The Criminal Justice System and alternatives approaches to treatment. These alternative approaches assist the reader in accepting that treatment programs can offer a variety of approaches to rehabilitation and healing. BC Partners can be contacted at phone number 1-800-661-2121; 604-669-7600; email bc-partners@heretohelp.bc.ca; web: www.heretohelp.bc.ca. Mailing address: Visions Editor, c/0 1200 – 1111 Metcalfe Street, Vancouver, BC V6E 3V6.

Victoria Maxwell is a Mental Health Educator, Consultant, Actor and Writer. She is a person diagnosed with Bipolar Disorder (Manic Depression) who provides leadership and inspiration to others struggling with their Mental Illness. On her "Crazy for Life" website her biography states the following: *"Victoria Maxwell is one of North America's most sought-after educators and consultants on the 'livid' experience of Mental Illness and recovery, early detection of depression, reducing stigma and creating corporate mental health strategies. After her diagnosis of bipolar* *disorder (Manic Depression) and psychosis, she became extremely proactive in her recovery process. She combines her theatre background, personal experience of psychiatric illness and professional knowledge as a group facilitator and mental health worker, to give a unique and powerful 'insider's' perspective on dealing with depression and other Mental Illnesses. Her company, Crazy for Life Co. assists organizations to enhance workplace wellness and return to work practices, recognize depression, and affect corporate mental 'wealth' action plans. Her most popular wellness package combines her solo show, Crazy for Life, with a customized workshop or keynote speech for either in-house training or a company conference. Creating Optimism: Recognizing Workplace Depression and Work Wise: Maintaining Mental Health without Going Crazy proves to be exceptionally inspirational and informative seminars and keynotes for companies and conferences across Canada. Talks focusing on creativity, presentation skills, storytelling, humour, writing and applied theatre are also available."*[5]

Victoria Maxwell, through her determination and commitment to increase public awareness and assist organizations, corporations, and individuals in reducing the stigma surrounding Mental Illness, not only "hears the silent voices" but speaks out for those who are not able to speak for themselves. Her vigilance and compassion also encourages those with silent voices to find their voices and make them heard. One person *can* make a difference in the world, and as Victoria Maxwell carries her message throughout North America and overseas, the demand for her consultation and seminars increases. On her website the following quotes appear: "Facts and Stats: Mental Illnesses are

caused by complex interplay of genetic, biological, personality, environmental factors. Canadian Mental Health
Association, 2005", "Odds and Ends: My only advice to stay
aware, listen carefully, and yell for help if you need it. Judy
Blume (author)." Victoria Maxwell continues to speak and
advocate for so many others; we are blessed to have her in
our lives! Further information can be obtained through her
website: www.victoriamaxwell.com.

There are countless organizations that further the cause
of public awareness of mental health issues throughout
North America. In Canada, the **Canadian Mental Health
Association** is known for updating the public on Mental
Illness. It plays an active role in lobbying politicians on the
federal level to influence public policy. "CMHA promotes
and advocates through strong connections with policy-
makers, mental health consumers and their families, educators, the media, stakeholders and other Service Providers.
Their national office influences public policy at the federal
level with a multifaceted approach that includes strength-
ening their relationship with governmental officials and
politicians. They also focus on the ongoing submission
of briefs and presentations to Standing Committees on
Finance, Health, Human Resources Development, Justice
and others".6 A person can access their position papers on
their website or write to their mail address for copies.

This organization is critical in connecting the concerns
and problems of people with Mental Illness to the decision
makers in our country who determine policies arising out
of federal legislation. These policies may be in the areas of
education, employment, health, research, and social services amongst others, and determine in part what programs

are funded to the provinces across the country. CMHA is a strong, political voice for persons who find it hard to express their needs and desires; it is an important national organization that updates the public on current research findings and policy initiatives presented to governmental officials. Its focus on understanding Mental Illness and coordinating the efforts of many individuals and various groups in order to present policy briefs and submissions to decision makers goes a long way to maintaining and acquiring new services for those with Mental Illness.

CMHA can be reached at the following address:

Canadian Mental Health Association
180 Dundas Street West, Suite 2301,
Toronto, Ontario, Canada
M5C 1Z8
Phone # 416-484-7750
Email: General enquiries: info@cmha.ca
Web site inquires: webmaster@cmha.ca

The Mood Disorders Association of British Columbia, Canada is a province-wide non-profit society built on a foundation of inclusion, compassion, and integrity. Its mission is as follows:

"The mission of the Mood Disorders Association of British Columbia is to provide support and education for people with a mood disorder, their families and friends as we build an understanding community. We will follow our mission statement by adhering to the following Philosophy Statements:

149

We celebrate our partnerships with individuals, their families, professionals and agencies. We believe in, value and respect:

- *the potential of each individual*

- *understanding, empathy, and listening as the cornerstone of self-help*

- *sharing and caring as a basis for healing*

- *honesty, trust and confidentiality*

- *inclusiveness, fellowship and hope*

- *the equality of all members in democratic, participative decision making*

- *the choices of individuals taking responsibility for their actions*

- *honest, non-judgmental support to individuals and families*

- *the contributions of individuals, their families and friends*

- *the skills of professionals and their role in recovery and support*

- *learning and self-awareness as part of the educative process*

- *research as part of best treatment and recovery[7]*

Many years ago, after Brent was first diagnosed, he suggested to me that we form a self-help support group in our community, Langley, B.C. Robert Winram, MDA's executive director at the time, provided us with much needed guidance and direction. Through MDA we were given educational resources, videos, and guest speakers to assist us in our weekly meetings. We also attended several MDA meetings where we shared ideas with others, met with resource persons involved in mental health issues, and received MDA's endorsement when we applied for a government grant for our group. This grant allowed us to buy a T.V., V.C.R., educational videos, and storage cabinet. We held many sessions with the aid of this equipment which included Persons with Mental Illness, their friends, and family members. Guest speakers updated us on research projects, medications, and other resources available through MDA.

When we attended the MDA meetings I was very impressed with the way in which Persons with Mental Illness were encouraged to participate in discussions and decision-making. The structure of the board includes Persons with Mental Illness along with Supporters and resource persons; each member has equal say in discussions, planning sessions and decisions made by the board. This has not changed over the years. MDA organizes education meetings, socials and fund raisers, "Highs and Lows" choir, provides guidance to self-help groups, young adults and families across the province and encourages the formation of new groups. Facilitator training is offered on a regular basis to those expressing an interest in leading one of these groups. Their regular newsletter contains poetry and letters from Persons with Mental Illness, lists of self-help group contacts, articles on mental health, current research projects, mental health information line numbers, letter from the editor, requests for feedback and opinions, and links to resources on Mental Illness.

One of MDA's goals, "reduce the sense of disgrace experienced by people with Mental Illness", is reflected in the warmth and compassion shown to anyone who walks in the office for information and support. The office is situated close to public transit in Vancouver and encourages people to drop in and access available resources. The staff and volunteers work hard as a team to reach out to those who seek assistance and are open to suggestions and ideas on how to improve and access resources. MDA provides links to other organizations such as HOPE: Helping Overcome Psychosis Early; Child and Adolescent Bipolar Foundation, B.C. Partners for Mental Health and Addictions Information, amongst others. MDA also keeps us up to date on plays, short stories, and books written by Persons with Mental Illness, Supporters, and resource persons. One can purchase educational videos through MDA when running support groups and/or workshops, seminars, and conferences on mental health issues.

Mood Disorders Association of B.C. plays a pivotal role in changing society's attitude towards Mental Illness from a negative, fearful one to that of increased understanding and willingness to participate in inclusive support programs. Persons with Mental Illness, in partnership with Service Providers and Supporters continue to contribute to the growth of resources and services offered through MDA.

MDA can be contacted as follows:

#202, 2250 Commercial Drive, Vancouver, B.C. V5N 5P9; phone number 604-873-0103; mdabc@telus.net; www.mdabc.ca.

British Columbia Coalition of People with Disabilities is another provincial non-profit organization in Canada that represents people who are challenged by all types of disabilities in B.C. The Coalition's mandate is as follows:

"to raise public and political awareness around issues of concern to disability communities and to create change; to improve people with disabilities access to all aspects of our communities."

- *"We advocate with all levels of government to improve policies and attitudes that affect people with disabilities;*

- *Promote public awareness of disability issues through conferences, special projects and the media;*

- *Provide individual and group advocacy for people with disabilities;*

- *Serve on government panels and committees;*

- *Share information and self-help skills with people with disabilities and disability organizations"*[8]

The **Coalition** plays a key role in lobbying policy and decision makers in our province, and their political influence continues to affect positive change. There are numerous examples of their influence on change in direction on pol-

153

icy initiatives in services for persons with disabilities.

I want to emphasize one example of political action that points out how a regressive change in government policy regarding eligibility for disability benefits caused undue hardship to thousands of persons applying for and/or renewing their benefits with the provincial government. The government at that time decided to tighten up eligibility criteria for those requesting assistance with the intent of reducing costs by literally cutting off many people from their disability income. One of the bureaucratic ways to do just that was the introduction of an application form (over 20 pages) that had to filled out by the applicant with detailed explanation (based on checklists) of why they required financial assistance. They had a limited time to fill out the form and get the signatures of those healthcare professionals involved in their treatment. Needless to say, the form was designed in such a way that it was very difficult for people to fill out; the criteria for receiving assistance eliminated almost everyone with a disability unless they were so disabled that they could barely function. Brent became emotionally immobilized when he saw the form and could not complete it without my assistance due to the stress it created. I read through it carefully and became very upset as I felt that the provincial government had no intentions of assisting those with disabilities. It was a cost cutting measure, consistent with their other policies to reduce public services and move towards privatization of healthcare.

The **Coalition** took on this issue — the executive director, **Margaret Burrell**, her staff, and board members "heard the silent voices" and organized an education and protest campaign that could not be ignored. Once the citizens of British Columbia gained a better understanding of the government's intentions, the **Coalition** had the ear of the politicians and was instrumental in pressuring the government to reverse its "reduce the numbers on disability" policy.

Other organizations working with persons with disabilities took up the fight as well until the government backed down. The government of the day had to save face as always but the end result meant continued financial assistance for those who needed it. Of course, the amount of financial assistance is never enough (below the poverty line), even though recently it was raised slightly by the provincial government. In addition, the **Coalition,** along with other organizations, has been instrumental in lobbying policy makers in government to increase the amount of earned income exemptions for those who are able to engage in gainful employment.

Networking by of the **Coalition** has created a much stronger coordination of education, advocacy, and services offered by several non-profit organizations in B.C. Persons with disabilities are included in day-to-day activities, planning sessions, and presentations on panels, public forums, and government committees. I appreciate the positive, direct approach taken by the **Coalition.** This organization provides constructive criticism and gives credit where due. For example, the **Coalition** makes the following comments pertaining to the federal government Disability Tax Credit: "The **BCCPD** and **BC Public Interest and Advocacy Centre (BCPIAC)** are pleased with the changes implemented by the federal government on the Disability Tax Credit. The application form (T2201) was amended in 2004 and people with mental health disabilities may now find it easier to qualify for the DTC. People with physical disabilities may also find it easier to access the DTC because of the changes. We have therefore concluded our campaign on this issue and would like to thank everyone who has shown support and helped us in this victory."[8]

BC Coalition of People with Disabilities can be contacted as follows:

> #204 – 456 West Broadway, Vancouver, B.C. V5Y 1R3; phone number 604-875-0188; TTY 604-875-8835; Email: feedback@bccpd.bc.ca.

The **BCPIAC**, as mentioned above, on behalf of a coalition of fifteen community groups, including the **Coalition**, provided leadership by filing a systemic complaint with the Ombudsman in February, 2006 about unfair practices experienced by people needing assistance from the provincial Ministry of Human Resources. Again, "hearing the silent voices", and speaking loudly not only to the public but through the court system is political action that affects positive change for so many.

Advocacy Access offered by the Coalition promotes economic rights advocacy for people with disabilities. In keeping with the goals and objectives of the Coalition this advocacy service concentrates in inclusion of all disabilities: mental health consumers, and people with physical, cognitive, and sensory disabilities. The Coalition's recent information states that Advocacy Access serves over 25,000 people a year. Its mandate is to:

- *Advocate on behalf of people with mental, physical, cognitive and sensory disabilities;*

- *Educate people with disabilities on their rights;*

- *Share self-help skills;*

- *Provide information on resources for people with disabilities;*

- *Provide referrals to community services for people with disabilities"*[8]

Specific economic areas include BC Employment and Assistance for Persons with Disabilities applications, re-considerations and tribunals, Schedule C health benefits, CPP Disability Benefits, Homeowner Grant for People with Disabilities, information on subsidized housing. The advocates walk people through the bureaucratic red tape, and provide support and advice in preparation for appeals, if necessary. The resource materials also available include, but are not limited to, help sheets, application guides, appeal guides, brochures, pamphlets, and advocacy manuals free of charge.

BC Coalition of People with Disabilities connects us to national programs by informing us of the activities of national groups such as The **Council of Canadians with Disabilities (CCD)**, decisions of various Human Rights Commissions throughout Canada as well as the **Canadian Human Rights Commission**. The **Coalition** has a wide base of funding which helps to ensure its ongoing work and includes many different groups, all dedicated to improving the lives of persons with disabilities. Its' voice is strong; its message is clear; and its dedication is relentless.

In my province, British Columbia, Canada, the **BC Human Rights Code** is legislation that **"recognizes that all persons are equal in dignity, rights and responsibilities, regardless of race, colour, ancestry, place of origin, age, sex, physical or mental disability, sexual orientation, religion, marital or family status, political belief and criminal convictions unrelated to the employment."**9 In terms of employment of persons with mental disabilities, the **duty to accommodate** is a legal requirement arising out of human rights legislation and case law in Canada. The case law is ever evolving as Employers, Unions, and Human Rights Commissions throughout Canada address, through the court system, the application of duty to accommodate to specific cases. It is important to note the following, as pointed out by the BC Human Rights Coalition:

"Although duty to accommodate is not found in the BC Human Rights Code, a series of Supreme Court of Canada decisions confirm the duty exists and applies to all provincially regulated employers. Where a barrier exists, or a policy or practice has adverse consequences on an individual in a protected group, the law says that the employer should reasonably accommodate that individual's difference provided they can do so, without incurring undue hardship, or without sacrificing a bona fide or good faith requirement of the job.

Undue hardship: Courts have determined that accommodation efforts must go to the point of undue hardship. While 'hardship' on its own infers a degree of effort is required, the threshold as to undue hardship is actually quite high. However, once an employer reaches that point, their legal duty to accommodate may be discharged. Factors that are used by the courts to assess the threshold include: financial costs; health and safety risks; and size and flexibility of the workplace. While a successful resolution to an accommodation request will vary greatly from one employer to another, more than mere inconvenience or disruption is expected in all situations."[10]

The **BC Human Rights Coalition** provides guidance for employers and those seeking accommodation. If an employee belongs to a Union, they can access the services of their Union in seeking accommodation. Unions and employers often cooperate through a joint Union/management process to assist an employee in returning to work after a period of illness and/or injury and accommodation may be granted at that time. Unions may also assist their members through the arbitration process in cases where there is no joint process or the joint process has not resolved the situation. Employees who do not belong to a Union can access the services of the **BC Human Rights Coalition** if their own efforts to seeking accommodation are unsuccessful.

Educational opportunities are offered by the **BC Human Rights Coalition** across British Columbia; this organization cooperates with community groups, employers, Unions, Colleges and others in delivering workshops that address the Human Rights Code and application of such in the workplace. Their website provides fact sheets, guidelines and policies on Duty to Accommodate with regular updates on recent court decisions. The application of the Supreme Court of Canada decisions on duty to accommodate continue to be tested by the court process as different perspectives on issues such as undue hardship, health and safety risks, and size and flexibility of workplaces may prevent satisfactory resolutions through the joint union/management process.

The **Ontario Human Rights Commission** provides an extensive manual on Policy and Guidelines on Disability and the Duty to Accommodate. This manual includes summaries of various court decisions and elaborates on issues such as undue hardship, removing barriers for persons with disabilities including physical, attitudinal and systemic ones, equal access to employment, etc. In their manual they make reference to **The United Nations' Declaration of the Rights of Disabled Persons**, declared in 1975, sections 3 and 8. "Disabled persons have the inherent right to respect for their human dignity. Disabled persons, whatever the origin, nature and seriousness of their handicaps and disabilities, have the same fundamental rights as their fellow citizens of the same age, which implies first and foremost the right to enjoy a decent life, as normal and full as possible; disabled persons are entitled to have their special needs taken into consideration at all stages of economic and social planning". This declaration sets the foundation on which society throughout the world can build human rights legislation and programs that flow out of this legislation.

The **Ontario Human Rights Commission** takes the view that accommodation in a job other than the pre-disability job may be appropriate in some circumstances and pursues the concept of temporary and permanent alternative work. For example, in terms of Mental Illness, the **Commission** makes the following statement:

"Mental Illness should be addressed and accommo-dated in the workplace like any other disability. In some cases, an employer may be required to pay special attention to situations that could be linked to mental disability. Even if an employer has not been formally advised of a mental disability, the perception of such a disability will engage the protection of the Ontario Human Rights' Code. Prudent employers should try to offer assistance and support employees before imposing severe sanctions. It should be borne in mind that some Mental Illnesses may render the employee incapable of identifying his or her needs.

Example: John has bipolar disorder, which he has chosen not to disclose to his employer because he is concerned about how he would be treated at work if it were known that he had a mental disability. He experi-ences a crisis at work, followed by a failure to appear at work for several days. The employer is concerned about John's absence and recognizes that termination for failure to report to work may be premature. The employer offers John an opportunity to explain the situation after treatment has been received and the situation has stabilized. Upon learning that a med-ical issue exists, the employer offers assistance and accommodation."[11]

The role of Supporter here is crucial as a liaison between the employee and employer. The Supporter may be the Union steward, Union staff representative on the joint union/management committee, Union representative or a friend and/or family member if the employee's worksite is not unionized. The Supporter can assist the employee in acquiring the necessary documents from medical professionals which often include recommendation for accommodation on the workplace as well as a gradual return to work program.

The **Commission** also points out that "those persons with disabilities are not necessarily required to disclose private or confidential matters, and should disclose information to the accommodation provider only as it pertains to the need for accommodation and any restrictions or limitations. Maintaining confidentiality for individuals with Mental Illness may be especially important because of the strong social stigmas and stereotyping that still persist about such disabilities."[11]

It is very encouraging for those persons with disabilities who are seeking accommodation on the workplace to be backed by the Supreme Court of Canada's decision as it pertains to undue hardship. "One must be wary of putting too low a value on accommodating the disabled. It is all too easy to cite increased cost as a reason for refusing to accord the disabled equal treatment." The cost standard is now, therefore, a high one based on the Supreme Court's decision. The Commission explains that "costs will amount to undue hardship if they are: quantifiable; shown to be related to the accommodation; and so substantial that they would alter the essential nature of the enterprise, or so significant that they would substantially affect its viability. This test will apply whether the accommodation will benefit one individual or a group. The costs that remain after all costs, benefits, deductions and other factors have been considered will determine undue hardship".

The Supporter can also alert the employer that sometimes outside sources of funding are available to the employee and employer to help cover costs of the accommodation, such as those provided by government programs, the employee's disability insurance, and other community services.

Human Rights Coalitions and Commissions, in general, focus on educating the public on their basic human rights, and advise on how to access court procedures to test the application of these rights in the workplace and in one's personal life. The Supporter can benefit from updating themselves on current cases before the courts, recent legal decisions, and resources available to assist persons with disabilities in fighting for their rights.

The **National Alliance on Mental Illness (NAMI), United States of America**, is the U.S.A.'s largest grassroots mental health organization dedicated to improving the lives of persons living with serious Mental Illness and their families. NAMI states that they are "dedicated to the eradication of Mental Illnesses and to the improvement of the quality of life of all whose lives are affected by these diseases." Their mission includes support, education, advocacy, and research for people living with Mental Illness.

What does NAMI do?

Public Education and Information Activities

- *www.nami.org – website which receives over 5.4 million visitors a year who turn to NAMI for information, referral, and education;*

- *888.999.6264 – toll-free Help Line serves over 4,000 callers a month and is staffed by a dedicated team of volunteer associates, as well as state and affiliate Help Lines in communities across the country;*

- *Public awareness activities such as Mental Illness Awareness Week, held during the first week of October, helps dispel the stigma surrounding Mental Illness and encourage early intervention and treatment;*

- *In Our Own Voice – available in selected communities across the country, this educational speakers bureau is presented by trained consumers living with Mental Illness to groups from all aspects of the community and both educates the public and supports consumer recovery and empowerment while dispelling the stigma of Mental Illness.*

Family and Consumer Peer Education and Support Activities

- *NAMI education programs include: Family-to Family, Provider Education Program, Peer-to Peer, and other state and local programs offered by trained family and consumer teachers to help educate other families, consumers, and professionals;*

- *Support groups offered through NAMI's 1100 affiliates in communities throughout the U.S.A.;*

Advocacy on Behalf of People Living with Mental Illness and for the Health of our Communities

- *NAMI advocates on the federal level to ensure non-discriminatory and equitable federal and private-sector policies are in place as well as a commitment to research for the treatment and cures for Mental Illness;*

- *NAMI's Campaign for the Mind of America, a grass-roots political communications initiative, focuses on building relationships at national, state, and local levels with community leaders and elected officials to ensure that policy decisions are reflective of the best economic, science, recovery, and systems choices while ensuring the best outcomes;*

- *NAMI's Action Centers, including the Multicultural Action Center, the Children & Adolescent Action Center, and the Center on Law and Criminal Justice, works to address unique systems and populations by developing, promoting, and disseminating appropriate education, advocacy, research, and support models tailored to meet specific needs.*

Public Events that raise funds and awareness while engaging the public, including:

- *NAMI Walks, NAMI's signature event, where thousands of concerned citizens in more than 50 communities across the U.S.A. will Walk for the Mind of America to raise money and awareness about the country's need for a world-class treatment and recovery system for people with Mental Illness;*

- *Unmasking Mental Illness Science and Research*

Gala, NAMI's annual black tie event held each fall in Washington, DC to raise funds and awareness for NAMI's efforts and to promote research into the causes and cures for Mental Illness."[12]

This nation-wide advocacy organization assists U.S. citizens in obtaining specific information on mental health programs and services in their particular state and/or community and provides links to other related organizations that also deal with mental health issues. As an umbrella group, NAMI is instrumental in educating and updating the American public on changes in legislation, research projects, and treatment programs available to those with Mental Illness.

Another national program, **The Carter Center Mental Health Program** was founded in 1991 by Mrs. Rosalynn Carter, who was awarded the Surgeon General's Medallion, (the only honor presented to civilians by the Surgeon General in the U.S.A.) for her outstanding leadership, advocacy, and commitment to improving the lives of those with Mental Illness. The Carter Center Mental Health Program focuses on four strategic goals:

"to reduce stigma and discrimination against people with Mental Illness; to achieve equity for mental health care comparable to other health care; to advance promotion, prevention, and early intervention services for children and their families; to increase public awareness worldwide about mental health and Mental Illness and to stimulate local actions to address those issues."[13]

At the international level, Mrs. Carter chairs the **International Committee of Women Leaders for Mental Health of the World Federation for Mental Health**, consisting of Royalty, Heads of State, and First Ladies. Detailed description of this organization's outreach work worldwide is available by contacting them as follows:

> The Carter Center
> One Copenhill
> 453 Freedom Parkway
> Atlanta, GA. 30307
> Phone # 404-420-5100
> E-mail address: carterweb@@emory.edu
> Website: www.cartercenter.org.[14]

The Global Alliance of Mental Illness Advocacy Networks, GAMIAN, is a not-for-profit international organization (non-political and non-sectarian) with its headquarters in New York City, concerned about mental health. **GAMIAN** is committed to the following:

> *"Empowerment of consumers to seek appropriate professional healthcare treatment for Mental Illness without fear of social stigma and with the recognition that such appropriate treatment will improve the quality of life of patients, their families, and their communities. GAMIAN is committed to promoting awareness of the constantly evolving knowledge abut the causes, consequences, and treatments of Mental Illness".*[15]

GAMIAN can be reached through their website: <u>www.gamian.org</u>.

It becomes evident that organizations involved in mental health issues, whether they be local, provincial, state, national, and/or international have similar mission statements, goals and objectives. They are a critical part of the evolving awareness and acceptance of those with Mental Illness by the rest of society. Education, research, treatment, recovery, support groups, social services, and employment programs are their focus as they strive to reduce the stigma of Mental Illness in society.

There are other organizations too numerous to include in this book. They can be reached by contacting those mentioned in this chapter. These organizations are also committed to improving the lives of Persons with Mental Illness and need secure funding to continue their education and advocacy programs.

Networking, building alliances, providing funds for necessary treatment, recovery, and support services allows the silent voices not only to be heard but encourages and supports them to speak up for themselves. The role of Supporter as advocate is carried out by countless persons throughout the world and is crucial to making sure the silent voices stay silent no more.

10

THROUGH THE EYES OF OUR SON

When I was born my eyes were wide open. According to my mother, I developed physically within the normal range but was a very serious infant who had a hard time smiling and laughing. I rolled over at three months, sat up at six months, crawled at seven months, and started to walk just before my first birthday. My parents were surprised that as early as seven months I would crawl over to bookshelves where I would organize the books. Although my speech development progressed, by the age of 2 my mother detected that I may be hard of hearing. Medical tests validated her concerns and I had surgery to correct the problem. However, I still have some hearing loss in my left ear to this day.

During pre-school years I learned how to dress myself, tie my shoes and ride a tricycle. I spoke in full sentences, enjoyed drawing and making figures out of Plastercene. During those years I stayed home most of the time with my parents and sister while attending part-time daycare, pre-school when I was 4 years old, and kindergarten when I turned 5. Apparently, I related and socialized well with other children, and was protective towards my sister.

We lived in a cold climate in Edmonton, Alberta at that time and skating and tobogganing were the main leisure activities in the winter. I was fascinated with dinosaurs and animals, and visited the Alberta Game Farm with my family on several occasions. During the summer we went camping, fishing, and took family vacations to visit relatives.

I recall little of what I felt during the early years. My mother became concerned when I found it hard to go to sleep, but still had energy for the next day. When I was 5, I started to withdraw from friends and wanted to play by my-self more frequently. This behaviour was the subtle signs of mania and severe depression. However, no one in the fam-ily or outside the family understood that I had the bipolar condition. I did live in a structured environment with both parents raising me until my parents separated and then divorced when I was 6 years of age. My life dramatically changed when they announced the divorce at that time.

From the age of 6 to 12, there was a lot of turmoil in my life. My family moved several times; sometimes I lived with my father, and other times with my mother and my sister. I managed to do well in my grades at school despite instabil-ity. When I turned 9, my mother met Bob, who had two chil-dren of his own. My mother and Bob joined their families and I was raised most of the time after that by both of them. I shifted my leisure activities from clay modeling and artistic projects to learning and participating in different sports.

My earliest recall of the bipolar condition was at 6 years of age in Edmonton, Alberta. I remember experiencing very high emotions one moment, and then crashing to a low depressive mood shortly afterwards. I did not understand what was happening to me and there was no one to tell me that what I was experiencing was normal or abnormal. As the years went by, I was sent to several Psychiatrists to pinpoint the problem but they were not able to come up with a diagnosis of the bipolar condition. Their ignorance and lack of proper education pertaining to Mental Illnesses in general resulted in passing off the emotional roller coast ride and strange behaviors' as the consequence of changing educational institutions, changing friends, and the instability caused by moving to different residences.

When I was 11 years old, my natural father had a nervous breakdown near Christmas of that year, and my mother decided to send my sister and me to live with my paternal grandparents in Ottawa in order to keep us safe. My sister returned home after two months but I stayed for six months. It was not a good idea for me to have been there as I buried the pain of my dad's breakdown and didn't receive any help to deal with it. On the outside, I appeared to be normal to everyone and did well in school and in sports. During those years I struggled many times with extreme high and low moods swings that I kept hidden from those around me.

Spiritually speaking, everyone in my immediate family was unbelievers. My natural father introduced me to eastern religions and to chanting. My mother didn't Influence me at all towards any religion and neither did my stepfather. When I turned 20, I remembered then my earlier religious conversion. I was 8 years old, sitting on a log at a beach In Vancouver with two other boys. A man walked up to me and with a serious look in his eyes told me that I was a sinner, but that Jesus loved me. He gave me a simple sinner's prayer to invite Jesus into my heart. I bowed my head and asked Jesus to be my Saviour. Immediately my heart flooded with God's love. It was so supernatural; I could only explain It as being In heaven with Jesus for a moment In time. I told my parents and sister about Jesus. However, I didn't understand my salvation and quickly fell away from the faith.

The adolescence years, ages 13 to 18, resulted In emotional breakdowns, many psychiatrist appointments, and no diagnosis of the bipolar condition. During Grade 8, I became obsessed with academics and sports. At the Awards Ceremony at school I received a trophy and scholarship for the highest academic and athletic standing for that grade. This obsession continued, leading to burnout, and although I managed to pass Grade 9 with high marks, I had to leave school two months early due to a major nervous breakdown. I recovered from that breakdown on my own during the summer months and returned to school where, again, I escaped into sports. I lived with my natural father for a few months In Grade 10 but returned to my mother's home when he showed manic, delusional behaviour. His behaviour during my preadolescent and adolescent years confused me even more as to what was wrong with me.

I developed a strong interest in bowling during those years. I started with my participation in a 5 pin Youth Bowling Council League In my community when I was sixteen years old. This resulted in a 176 average, and the following year my average improved to 206 which was the highest average in the league. I discovered 10 pin bowling next, and I also competed in baseball, basketball, hockey, football, tennis, soccer, badminton, volleyball and track and field. My best time for the 1500 metre race at age sixteen was 4:26 minutes.

I did not rebel during adolescence. Sometimes, I engaged in excessive drinking on the weekends but did not use drugs or participate in sex. From grades 9 to 12, my best friend, Rob, and I would skip school frequently. I applied little effort to academics during the last two years of high school but somehow, managed to graduate from high school at age 18.

From infancy to age 18 I was able to function in the world quite well despite disturbing manic and depressive moods. Psychiatrists pointed out that moving constantly; changing schools and making new friends caused a lot of stress and instability in my life. However, a diagnosis of Mental Illness was not given.

After I graduated from high school, my natural father and I moved into a townhouse complex in Surrey, B.C. My father was owner, editor, and publisher of Life Gazette newspaper. For a few months, I drove to people's homes whose addresses were listed in church directories and sold subscriptions to Life Gazette. Door to door soliciting to sell items for Cobra Imports came next, followed by door to door canvassing of Sooter's photography portraits. A friend of mine had a father who was manager of Dare Foods cookie factory so I was able to get a job packaging cookies on an assembly line.

At that time, one of my friends from high school, Steve, invited me to Countyline Christian Fellowship Church in Aldergrove, B.C. for a youth service. It was there that the Lord met me again in a very powerful fashion, manifesting his love and forgiveness in my life. Praise and worship stirred my soul to the point of tears as I confessed Jesus as Lord of my life. The following day, repentance followed as I destroyed all my possessions that were ungodly. I stopped seeing un-believing friends and became friends with other Christians.

My terrible habit of swearing was completely gone.

I had expressed to the pastor of Countyline Church, George, that I would like to attend Bible College, He and his wife, Edith, offered their basement suite rent-free while I attended College so I moved out of my father's apartment and moved into his suite.

During my childhood years, the mania was short-lived, and really showed its ugly face when I was 19 years old. During my first year at Bible College I did not realize that I was manic. I was involved in street ministry, bible study fellowship, and studying my courses. This resulted in little down time. The only awareness that I had was that I had excessive energy.

After I attended my first year of college at Western Pentecostal Bible College (full-time from 1988-1989), I acquired a full-time summer job at Richmond Teen Challenge - a program where I worked as a youth counselor in a residential home for young offenders. Unfortunately, I experienced a traumatic Incident with one of the teenagers who held a knife to my throat and threatened to kill me. I thought I was going to die. I believe that this incident triggered the downside of my bipolar condition. When the summer was over, I returned to my second year at Bible College but had to withdraw due to severe depression.

Then the mania took over. I ended up the streets of Vancouver where I preached the gospel to people who were homeless. In a state of delusion with racing thoughts and chronic insomnia, it took several months for me to come down off the mania. Periods of sleep deprivation for 40-70 hours were common. Fortunately, no-one attacked me while I walked and ran through the streets of Vancouver all day and night (in dangerous areas such as Main and Hastings, and Cordova Street).

Finally, I was hospitalized at Langley Memorial Hospital and diagnosed by a Psychiatrist as having Bipolar Affective Disorder. I was 21 years old and stayed in Hospital for three and ½ months. This was the beginning of a slow and painful recovery process that lasted for almost two years.

After I withdrew from Bible College and following my hospitalization, I was only able to hold down part-time employment for short periods of time because my mood swings did not allow me to sustain regular employment. Several short term jobs ended because of my depression or employers "letting me go", probably because they didn't understand and couldn't deal with my manic episodes.

In 1994, I received a government grant to attend British Columbia Institute of Technology (BCIT), and registered in the full-time radio broadcasting program. It was a four year degree condensed into two years; the stress load was so high that I went in to full blown mania in January of the following year. I became incapable of attending BCIT and gravitated towards the streets of Vancouver. While I lived on the streets, I had incredible energy, my emotions were magnified, and, again, used my passion for evangelizing by sharing the good news of Jesus Christ with as many people as possible. I found myself mostly walking although I did run for several hours in a day. Typically I would not sleep for 40 to 70 consecutive hours, then sleep for 2 to 4 hours, and continue the sleep deprivation cycle all over again.

In all the years of mania, I was only physically assaulted in the face once in a bar in downtown Vancouver and I did not feel any physical pain from the assault.

The chemical imbalance in my brain caused me to be extremely delusional, and I believed that I owned car dealerships, supermarkets and other businesses in Vancouver. Occasionally I would take merchandise from some places of business without paying for them because I believed I was the owner. I knocked on people's doors, asked for free merchandise and organized garage sales on the streets to earn money for food.

During my employment at Richmond Teen Challenge I had saved about $4,000 from my wages, and it did not take me long to spend this money by feeding the poor. Even when I was delusional I never hallucinated at any time and was always aware of my surroundings. On two separate occasions I met two different individuals that I thought were human, but when they both disappeared before my eyes, I realized that the Lord had sent holy angels to confirm that he loved me and was concerned about my state of health. For anyone who is interested in angelic visitations, there are many books that have been written about this subject. Despite those encounters and the positive advice that I received from people around me, I was so "possessed" by the mania, or "under the influence" of the mania that I was a different person than I am during periods of stability when my thinking and behaviour are normal.

During manic episodes I sometimes lose too much weight from not eating properly, getting little sleep, and running for long periods of time; the flipside of mania led to excessive weight gain. For several years, the medication, Lithium, stabilized me in Hospital, and eventually I was switched to a mood stabilizer, Divalproic Acid as well as Loxapine to control the mania. Hospitalizations lasted about five weeks and although people came in to visit me they were not able to help me fight the depression that always followed the mania. The days were filled with emptiness, despair, and darkness and it seemed like there was no one who had the ability to make a difference in the recovery process.

Throughout these years I have tried to pursue my interest in Biblical studies and managed to complete five courses offered by Liberty College of Ministries (part-time in the evenings) and one course at Columbia Bible College. Mania reared its ugly head after I completed my course at Columbia Bible College, and ended up in hospital again. From 1991, the year I was diagnosed with the bipolar condition to present, I have been hospitalized thirteen times, the last time being early 2004. Since 2004 I have struggled mostly with depression, but recently managed to complete two courses at Summit Bible College (formerly Western Pentecostal Bible College).

My memory of extreme high and low mood swings goes back as early as 6 years of age. It was a relief at age 21 to finally understand what was wrong with me.

There has been good that has come out of this Illness. In 1990 I started a support group for people with Mental Illness which was held on a regular basis in my community. I applied for and received a government grant off $6,000 which paid for a new television, V.C.R., cabinet, videos, literature on mental health issues and Mental Illness, and outings in the community. My mother and I led the support group for five years.

It has taken me twenty years to gain insight on how to properly manage this mood disorder. A high stress level must be avoided and sleep deprivation can trigger mania as well.

My last manic episode in 2004 resulted in a breakthrough. For the first time, I recognized the early warning signs of mania before full blown mania took over and agreed to admit myself into the Hospital. Many demons have been fought, but now there is reason to be more optimistic about my future years.

Could it be that during the most difficult times of a person's life there is nothing or little that anyone can do other than be a good listener and pray that it won't take too long before the severe depression passes? Cause and effect stipulates that the longer and more intense the mania is the longer and more intense the depression will be. As wonderful as mania can be at times, it is not worth it to experience the mania because the consequences are too severe. Therefore, taking your medication daily, being honest with your Psychiatrist and your support team is crucial in preventing the mania from happening in the first place. The warning signs I look for are sleep deprivation and not feeling fatigued afterwards, excessive energy, and constantly talking. If you experience consistent stress for more than a week then you should reconsider reducing or eliminating what you believe is causing the stress in the first place. Too much stress will eventually trigger a hypo-manic state which then ultimately leads to full-blown mania. Medications usually take several weeks before they make a difference in your life so you should see your Psychiatrist at least once a month to monitor the medications. Take your blood tests as directed by the Psychiatrist as it is necessary to check how your internal organs are responding to the medications.

There are simple steps that I take to try and prevent further episodes: exercise, eating properly, regular sleeping pat-

terns, taking medications daily, and time with family and friends.

After seeing God's hand in my life, especially his love and compassion in helping me recover from terrible and scary bouts of despair, there is no doubt in my mind that God can restore people regardless of their circumstances. The future years will be devoted to receiving a much deeper healing in my life so I can turn around and comfort people who are suffering like I have suffered all of my life. Recently I have been attending the Freedom Session Program in my community. This is a 12 step Christ centered program that focuses on healing and supporting one another. God has done some powerful healing through this program.

I believe that the most important thing is my relationship with Jesus Christ because God reveals the truth to you through the scriptures in the Bible. His presence gives you hope that somehow you will eventually have this condition under control and experience a higher quality of life.[16]

11

HOPE THROUGH COMPASSION AND DESPAIR

Hope is "the confident expectation that a desire will be fulfilled"; 17 the desire of the Supporter is to see their loved one acquire peace of mind through a meaningful life with themselves and others. The Supporter opens their heart with unconditional love and support and feels a connectedness to others who experience pain and suffering as they try so hard to cope with their Mental Illness. This connectedness is compassion; the pain and suffering the Supporter so often witnesses are their loved one's despair. The Supporter, even in their own darkest moments of frustration and sadness, must continue to nurture their inner spirit, as it is this spirit that sends rays of hope to those suffering from Mental Illness.

The chapter, **Letting Go**, emphasizes the importance of nurturing oneself, and points out how necessary it is to recharge one's emotional battery in order to provide support to others who are struggling and suffering with Mental Illness. "Hope springs eternal" when one remains true to themselves in their daily walk through life, as they map out a path to compassion and understanding. This compassion must be directed towards themselves as well — compassion for their own hardship, pain, and sadness as they watch others suffer so much, and compassion for themselves when they get frustrated and discouraged by their own efforts that don't seem to be helping the Person with Mental Illness. One's efforts may or may not have a direct impact on the life of someone else, but if these efforts are made without expectations there is a greater chance that they will be received by others as gestures of good will, rather than attempts to control and manipulate their lives.

It never fails to amaze me how other Supporters persevere in their efforts to assist and advocate for family members and/or friends who suffer from Mental Illness even when they, themselves, are coping with their own illnesses. "Lee" is a mother of four adult children whom I met many years ago when I lived in an intentional community. One of her sons was diagnosed with schizophrenia at the time that I met Lee and her family in the community and I recall how much I was moved by her determination to seek help and find resources to assist her son. My own son was only 9 years old and I had no idea that I would be facing the same challenges that Lee was dealing with so many years ago. There were few resources available and the stigma of Mental Illness was a major roadblock to public support and government funding for programs and services. I asked Lee recently what kept her going, and she stated that her own faith, through prayer and meditation, has renewed her spirit and commitment to stay connected to her son. She has persevered over the years by finding resources and advocating for her son when it is necessary.

Lee educated members of our intentional community on Mental Illness—the signs, symptoms, and struggles that both she and her son faced on a daily basis. Today, Lee, while struggling with her own stresses and Parkinson's disease, maintains regular contact with all her adult children and appreciates the ongoing support of her partner. As I sat in her living room, after so many years had gone by, I was impressed by her warmth, grace, and kind spirit. I felt a deeper sense of understanding for what both of us experience as mothers of sons who suffer from Mental Illness and appreciated her candor and interest in my life. Lee's positive acceptance of her situation and her tenacity to overcome new obstacles that present themselves shows other Supporters, including myself, that we can face adversity without losing our sense of self and purpose. I feel stronger after meeting her again, and only hope that this renewed strength will be passed on to others in my journey.

As I look back on my days on a communal farm, I will never forget one of the community members, John, a single parent of two girls at the time, one of whom was in a wheelchair due to her physical disability. She was able to walk briefly with braces and would come out to the farm with her father for workdays and/or farm meetings. The first time I met John and his daughter; I couldn't help but be impressed with the way in which he related to her. He was patient, kind, and determined to assist her if she needed help, but her spirit and desire to be as independent as possible was amazing, to say the least. John, who was a dynamic leader in the community, related to his daughter as a person first. That taught so many of us who witnessed their relationship, that persons with disabilities have their own personalities, interests, desires, and dreams for their future. His daughter showed interest in our lives on the farm, and interacted well with our children, who also benefited from seeing her efforts to adapt and cope with the obstacles around her. I recall, during one visit, how John's daughter maneuvered her wheelchair down the steps of the farmhouse, and joined other children in their activities on the farm. She did not withdraw in the farmhouse and keep to herself; her delightful, positive energy radiated to those around her.

Over the years John continued to remain by her side, an advocate when necessary, and a devoted father. Just as I was touched by Lee's unconditional love for her son, I was also deeply moved by John's dedication to his daughter. My impression of their relationships to their children stayed with me, and helped me respond the same way to Brent. They were my mentors, without even knowing it, and I am truly thankful for having met them during that time of my life.

Another member of the intentional community, Murph, who still lives in the community at the writing of this book, was very kind recently to share her insights about her bipolar condition. Murph did not become afflicted with acute symptoms of manic-depression until she was in her 40's. She explained to me that although her life changed dramatically because of the illness she was able to live the first forty years of her life with stability, and felt that she had accomplished much during that time. It was incredible how Murph felt compassion for others, who did not have long periods of stability in their younger years, and thus,

were not able to look back on their achievements and relationships with some sense of success and fulfillment.

When I met Murph so many years ago I immediately
liked her, enjoyed her sense of humour, and admired her
concern for others who suffered from disabilities. Although
she was struggling with serious bouts of depression and
mania she showed concern for Brent, and helped me gain
some perspective on my situation. She listened intently,
offered suggestions, and understood what he was experiencing, which in turn, gave me a deeper comprehension of
what was happening in his mind. Murph cares for others
around her, and has contributed her time and energy into
building community. When I asked her where her support came from, if any, during her most difficult times,
she referred to an acute episode several years ago. She had
received psychiatric care in a Hospital for several weeks.
Murph recalled how several members of the community
formed a 24 hour support team around her, culminating
in assisting her to the Hospital, and visiting her during
her stay there. After Murph stabilized in the Hospital, she
returned to her community, and gained employment, assisting others with disabilities, until she retired. Recently
her life-long and closest friend passed away, causing her
grief and sadness that could easily have triggered another
acute episode. However, Murph managed to draw on her
inner strength and carry on. She appreciates living in community, rather than alone in isolation, and copes with not
only Manic-Depression, but Arthritis and Crohn's Disease.
Murph is a witty and intelligent woman, always interested
in my life, and so honest about her own. This honesty and
integrity is not only comforting to me but takes me to a

place where I feel introspective and peaceful after our conversations. Murph gives me Hope!

I also benefited during my career as a Union representative from my relationship with Patrice, a Director in our Union, who supervised me most of the time that I was Education Officer of my Union. Patrice, a single parent to her daughter who has Williams' Syndrome, is the epitome of a Supporter who gives unconditional love and support and advocates not only for her daughter but for many others who struggle with disabilities. I learned so much from her as she provided guidance and sound advice on how to access and advocate for programs and services. Patrice was, and continues to be, a strong advocate—she is positive, assertive, and a skilled networker who acknowledges and values contributions that others make to improve the lives of people with disabilities.

Patrice was tenacious in working with the school system such that her daughter completed Grade 12, a tremendous accomplishment for a young person with Williams' Syndrome. Patrice's leadership role has showed other parents that they could lobby for and acquire educational resources for their children as well by networking with one another and cooperating with school administrators and school boards. Patrice taught me to consider different angles to solving a problem and showed me ways to remove, go around, and/or over obstacles when I was advocating for Brent. I learned from her how to be assertive (rather than aggressive), an invaluable skill as an advocate. I know that Patrice's leadership and dedication also helps other Supporters who continue to benefit from her own experiences and commitment to persons with disabilities.

Paula West, author of **"Just a Mom"**, writes of her personal journey through her daughter's Mental Illness. A summary of her book is outlined as follows:

> *"From the outside, Paula's life was ideal. The idyllic small town farm life, a husband, a comfortable home and four healthy children all seemed perfect to her neighbors and friends. The illusion shattered when her teenage daughter was diagnosed with a Mental Illness. In this true life story, Paula lets us into her world as she and her family struggle with the roller coaster life of a loved one with bipolar disorder, formerly known as Manic Depression. Told through Paula's eyes, we see her daughter fall deeper and deeper into despair and suicidal behaviors. We watch as her family tries to give their daughter and sister strength to live in the world. This story will make you believe in miracles and give you hope in the darkest of hours".* [18]

As I read each chapter of this book I was amazed at how similar the author's experiences were to those of my own. It was emotionally difficult for me to read her book at first, as it reminded me of my own journey and how much pain I had also suffered. Always trying to deal with the task at hand, I tried to overcome my own fears as to what lay ahead, and realized that Paula West, like so many other parents, did not give up her pursuit of finding out information on Mental Illness, providing unconditional love and support to her daughter, and advocating on her behalf when it was necessary. The author takes each step of her journey with optimistic caution and shows us how to live in the moment and cherish the times that you spend with those you love who are trying to cope with their Mental Illness. Her faith, like my own, has guided her through this difficult journey, and given her strength when she felt there was nothing left to give. Her deep sense of spirituality, love for her daughter and her family is evident as she tells the reader her story. "**Just a Mom**" clearly points out that "Mental Illness is a family disease; no one is left untouched by the loved one's distress. Lifestyle, emotional stability and financial resources become vulnerable victims. Regardless of their spiritual beliefs, family members may experience a crisis of faith as they attempt to understand why this is happening and how they can help".

I was especially touched by the dedication of her book to her daughter as she states:

> *"For Kristen, and all who live with a mental disorder. May you spend each day here on earth safe in the arms of the angels. Also, for Mom and Dad, Beth and all the "earth angels" who encouraged and supported us. Special thanks to Brian and my family, especially Kristen, who insisted that for the sake of mental health awareness our story must be told".*

I thank Paula West for sharing her experiences and educating her readers on the reality of Mental Illness as well as giving us information and resources available to those seeking help.

I am sure there are Supporters throughout the world, like those I have mentioned above, that persistently persevere on a daily basis with Mental Illness in their families.

Their stories may not have been told to others but many are witness to their commitment and strength as they try so hard to ease the suffering of the ones they love.

I often observe others in public who accompany someone with a disability. I never stop searching for ways to be more appropriate as I interact with persons with disabilities. Mental Illness is often an invisible disability which goes unnoticed unless a person is engaged in an acute episode of their illness. During those occasions where I have been witness to someone who is expressing signs of agitation, anxiety and/or panic, I immediately look to see if someone else is with them. I have been able to interact with "that someone" and offer my assistance by relating directly to the person who is agitated. There are times when I have helped by speaking to them directly in a calm, quiet manner, asking them if I can assist them with anything. One can also check out the location of security and management in public facilities if a person's behaviour appears to be a threat to themselves and/or others. Sometimes the immediate Supporter is preoccupied with the person who is experiencing an episode and cannot leave them to get assistance from others. It is not uncommon for bystanders to stand there and watch without offering assistance because they are not sure how to help. I encourage others to offer support to those in these awkward, stressful situations by acting towards them in an objective but compassionate manner.

I have been encouraged over the last few years by the increase of education programs in training sessions for Police Officers, Paramedical Personnel, and other Service Providers. These programs assist in providing the necessary tools for peaceful, compassionate intervention when Persons with Mental Illness are being overcome by their illness. This type of intervention often helps in providing medical care and other community supports on an emergency basis, and may defuse situations where a person suffering from an acute attack of their illness cannot control the acceleration of their symptoms. The more that education and training is provided to emergency response teams, the greater the chances that these personnel will show compassion and understanding during their intervention. This kind of intervention is critical for those who are mentally ill in order to decrease the trauma of intervention, and increase their trust level towards emergency responders who treat them with kindness and respect.

One can't help but be optimistic when programs, such as "**Moving Beyond**", aim at assisting young people (ages 17 to 29) with mental health issues. This program is offered by the **Mood Disorders Association of B.C.** and allows young people to support each other, even if they don't have an actual mental health diagnosis. One of the participants who has become a facilitator points out in **VISIONS**, BC's Mental Health and Addictions Journal, Summer, 2006 issue, the purpose of this support group for youth. "Each of us is on our own pathway to recovery, but we share the common bond of experiencing or suspecting what is known as a psychiatric experience. With our peers, we transition through different stages of recovery together. We have fun, learn to become aware, share our experiences through telling our stories and listening to one another, and build community together".[19]

The **Friends for Life Program**, developed in Australia,

is a world-leading early intervention and prevention program that aims to reduce the risk of anxiety disorders and builds resilience (emotional strength) in children. It helps children to identify the thoughts they have about themselves and others, and teaches them how to talk positively to themselves, as well as how to respond to body clues through awareness and relaxation activities, problem-solving, rewarding self and facing fears. This program is being offered to grades four and five students throughout the Province of British Columbia, in support of the Child and Youth Mental Health Plan for B.C.

The acronym '**FRIENDS**' stands for:

- *Feelings*

- *Remember to relax*

- *I can do it*

- *Explore solutions and coping step plans*

- *Now reward yourself! You've done your best!*

- *Don't forget to practice*

- *Smile. Stay calm.* [20]

Parents and Caregivers are also included in this program which helps them become aware of the tools and life skills that their children are learning through FRIENDS. The parents also learn how best to support their children in using these skills at home, and learn how to recognize and respond to signs of anxiety not only in their children, but also within themselves. Further information on this

innovative program can be found at <u>www.friendsinfo.</u>
<u>net/downloads/FRIENDS</u>.

Information, services, programs and research on Mental
Illness continue to progress as Supporters, organizations,
private and public institutions, and Persons with Mental
Illness strive to reduce and remove stigma, improve quality of life, and work towards a cure. It may seem at times
that despair is the order of the day, but compassion and
understanding will win in the end as we share our experiences for the common good.

As I come to the end of my story, I can only hope that
my experiences and suggestions will assist Supporters in
their journey towards understanding and assisting those
who struggle with Mental Illness.

Recently, Brent reunited with his natural father at our
Thanksgiving dinner, after so many years of being apart.
After I opened my door to welcome Brent's father into our
home we talked about old times and enjoyed each other's
company, sharing a common bond of love and concern
for our children. Then we sat down for dinner and Brent
said Grace, thanking God for our time together. He showed
kindness and warmth towards his father, and again, I was
overcome by his strength of character and loving nature.
Yes, there is Hope through Compassion and Despair.

REFERENCES

1. Canadian Mental Health Association pamphlet, **Who Turned out the Lights?,** Canadian Mental Health Association, #416-484-7750; 180 Dundas Street, Suite 2301, Toronto, ON M5G 1Z8; www.webmaster@cmha.ca.

2. Definition of ADVOCATE: Webster's Encyclopedia Dictionary of the English Language, Canadian Edition, 1988, Lexicon Publications, INC.

3. Reliable Business Outsourcing, www.reliable@southfraser.com, #604-864-5770, ext. 308, Toll-free:#1-877-827-8249.

4. **VISIONS,** B.C.'s Mental Health and Addictions Journal, BC Partners for Mental Health and Addictions, 1200-1111 Metcalfe Street, Vancouver, B.C. V6E 3V6; #1-800-661-2121; #604-669-7600; www.heretohelp.bc.ca.

5. **Victoria Maxwell,** Mental Health Educator, Consultant, Actor and Writer, www.victoriamaxwell.com.

6. Canadian Mental Health Association
180 Dundas Street West, Suite 2301
Toronto, Ontario, Canada
M5C 1Z8
#416-484-7750
webmaster@cmha.ca

7. Mood Disorder Association of B.C., #604-873-0103; #202, 2250 Commercial Drive, Vancouver, B.C. V5N 5P9; www.mdabc.ca.

8. B.C. Coalition of People with Disabilities, #604-875-0188
#204, 456 Broadway, Vancouver, B.C. V5Y 1R3; E-mail: feedback@bccpd.bc.ca.

9. BC Human Rights Code, B.C., Canada

10. BC Human Rights Coalition, #604-689-8474; Toll-free # 1-877-689-8474; contact email: info@bchrcoalition.org.

11. Ontario Human Rights Commission; #416-314-4500; 180 Dundas Street West, 8th Floor, Toronto, ON M7A 2R9; E-mail: info@ohrc.on.ca.

12. National Alliance on Mental Illness (**NAMI**), www.nami.org.

13. Carter Center Mental Health Program, The Carter Center, # 404-420-5100; One Copenhill, 453

Freedom Parkway, Atlanta, GA 30307
www.cartercenter.org.

14. International Committee of Women Leaders for
Mental Health of the World Federation for Mental
Health, www.cartercenter.org.

15. The Global Alliance of Mental Illness Advocacy
Networks (**GAMIAN**), www. gamian.org.

16. **Our Son's own words on his struggle with Mental
Illness; Through The Eyes of Our Son;**

17. **Definition of HOPE: Webster's Encyclopedic
Dictionary, Canadian Edition, 1988.**

18. **Paula West,** author, **Just a Mom**, Copyright
2001; Patio Publishing Company, Canada. E-mail:
paula948@hotmail.com.

19. **Moving Beyond**, program of Mood Disorders
Association of B.C.

20. **Friends for Life,**
www.friendsinfo.net/downloads/FRIENDS.

SUGGESTED READINGS

1. **Bipolar 11**, Ronald Fieve, RMD; Rodale Publishing Co., 2006

2. **Living Well with Depression & Bi Polar Disorder**, John McManamy, Collins Publishing Co., 2006

3. **Taking Charge of Bipolar Disorder**, Julie A. Fast & John Preston, PsyD.; Warner Wellness, Hachette Book Group USA, 2006

4. **Taming Bipolar Disorder**, Psychology Today, Lori Oliveenstein, Alpha Co., 2004

5. **Brilliant Madness, Living with Manic Depression**, Patty Duke & Gloria Hochman, Bantum Publishers, 1997

6. **Caring for the Mind, Comprehensive Guide to Mental Health,** Bantum Books, 1995

ISBN 142511697-3

9 781425 116972